The Undivided Self

Alexander Technique and the Control of Stress

THEODORE DIMON, Jr.

North Atlantic Books
Berkeley, California

The Undivided Self

Published by
North Atlantic Books
P.O. Box 12327
Berkeley, California 94712

Cover art by Legacy Media
Cover and book design by Legacy Media
Figures 2, 3, 4a, and 4b by Christine Gralapp, M.A.
Printed in the United States of America

The Undivided Self is sponsored by the Society for the Study of Native Arts and Sciences, a nonprofit educational corporation whose goals are to develop an educational and crosscultural perspective linking various scientific, social, and artistic fields; to nurture a holistic view of arts, sciences, humanities, and healing; and to publish and distribute literature on the relationship of mind, body, and nature.

Library of Congress Cataloging-in-Publication Data

Dimon, Theodore.
    The undivided self: Alexander technique and the control of stress /
Theodore Dimon, Jr.
        p. cm.
    Includes bibliographical references.
    ISBN 1-55643-294-1 (pbk. : alk. paper)
    1. Alexander technique.   I. Title.
BF172.D56   1998
615.8'2—dc21   98-18328
                                                                    CIP

1   2   3   4   5   6   7   8   9   /   03   02   01   00   99

To the transcendent inheritance of a conscious mind

For my father, Theodore Dimon, Sr., who taught me the true meaning of philosophy: the love of wisdom.

Table Of Contents

....

Foreword *by Walter Carrington*

This book is a unique and welcome contribution to the published literature on the work of F. Matthias Alexander. It is not an introduction or an exposition of his technique, but it offers the average intelligent reader an intellectual evaluation of his underlying principles and ideas.

Alexander defined his technique as a method of practical self-help, the outcome of his personal experience, based on the principle of Prevention and the recognition of the Unity of Mind and Body. He hoped that when its significance was fully appreciated, it would be taken up universally, and not be restricted to the benefit of any class or group of individuals, intellectuals or otherwise. Obviously, such a technique must be experienced before it can be understood; but as people gain practical experience of its application in their own lives, many thoughts and speculations about its implications inevitably arise.

First of all, they tend to regard it as a "treatment" or a "cure" or as some form of "somatic" education; and they preoccupy themselves with the practical requirements of "inhibition" or "withholding consent," and "direction," facilitating that relativity of the parts of the body on which poise and freedom of movement depend, the relativity that Alexander termed Primary Control. Only gradually do they come to appreciate its wider implications for life in general, particularly in the fields of psychology and education.

This is what Ted Dimon has sought to address in the following pages. He treats the concept of the use of the self, not in a restricted sense of the use of body and limbs in activity and movement, but comprehensively, including the brain, mind, thought, feeling, and emotion. For him, Alexander's most important discovery was the significance of our manner of use of ourselves, of how we use ourselves in daily life but also of how we could use ourselves differently if we chose to do so. He suggests that it is because people do not appreciate the true nature of their own problems, which stem mainly from a habitual and unrecognized misuse of themselves, that they find it difficult to see the significance of the principles on which the Technique is based.

He views tension and stress as among the most common problems of our daily life and shows how it is we ourselves, in our ignorance, who are the victims of our own misbehavior. He also shows how a change in our thinking and particularly a change in our preconceptions as to consciousness and the unity of mind and body could remedy the situation. Altogether he provides much food for thought in an area of human experience largely unexplored.

Walter Carrington
London
13 April 1998

Acknowledgments

I would like to express my gratitude to Walter and Dilys Carrington, my teachers and mentors; Professors Vernon Howard and Israel Scheffler, my graduate school advisors; Anne Panagakos, for her constant support; Jeremy Paul, for his critical reading of the manuscript and years of friendship; and Seymour Simmons, for his constant encouragement and support, as well as help with the illustrations.

I would also like to thank Jay Kramer, my lawyer and agent, who has made the publishing phase of this book so much easier than it might otherwise have been; Judy Dimon for her support and talent for getting things done; Kevin Cole for his invaluable advice on how to improve the manuscript; Michael Schaeffer for his editing suggestions; Emily Weinert for her help in the production of the book; and Richard Grossinger and North Atlantic Books.

Finally, I would like to express my gratitude to my grandparents Panos and Theonia Dimon; my mother, Themis Dimon; my father, Theodore Dimon, Sr., to whom this book is dedicated; and Dena Davis, my constant supporter, partner, and friend, without whom I might never have finished this book.

Introduction

All around us we are witnessing the emergence of a new paradigm in health and healing. In medicine, education, sports, and psychology, there is a search for a new approach to bodily health based on an increasing appreciation that health is not purely mechanical, that the mind influences the body, and that bodily health must be seen in the context of a larger holistic framework. Medicine is experiencing a return to the concept of wholeness. There is a renewed interest in old forms of healing that naturally gravitate toward techniques which are not strictly mechanistic. Many doctors now practice some form of alternative medicine and are willing to embrace less traditional ideas. And a proliferating literature is demonstrating scientifically the link of immune function and various illnesses with moods, emotions, and mental attitude.

Among the many fascinating aspects of this movement, there is perhaps no more promising feature than the concept of self-direction. Where once the doctor ministered to illness, now we take health into our own hands, in the form of relaxation, exercise, mind/body techniques designed to calm the mind, calm the body, calm the emotions, release tension, free movement, and so on. In short, we have claimed the mind and body as our own domain, and express this empowered approach to our health in the form of a profusion of methods for controlling and understanding it.

This development is neither a haphazard event in the history of thought, nor the result of a deliberate ideological effort to transcend the limitations of medicine or old thinking. The new, or renewed, interest in the mind/body relationship comes, very simply, out of the pressure of needing to solve simple problems for which medical science cannot account. Tension, backache, and various stress-related problems all manifest themselves in the form of medical symptoms; yet medicine as we have known it is simply not able to fully address these problems, which require not simply treatment but conscious understanding, awareness, and responsibility. Hence the growing trend toward self-help and awareness programs.

But the proliferation of methods which address this new set of problems has in many ways added to, not detracted from, the confusion about the subject—not just because of the sheer number of choices offered to the public, but because of the lack of clarity about exactly what the problems are. Methods for calming the system, for instance, have been shown to produce concrete results, thus demonstrating a direct link between mental states and physiology. Through meditation, it is possible to directly influence heart rate and metabolism. In short, these systems have demonstrated a clear ability to address various complex problems, by demonstrating a link between mind and body that has immediate uses and relevance.

But exactly what is the relation between the mind and body, why does consciousness play such an important role, and have we fully utilized the potential of conscious awareness? In virtually all the methods in current use today, consciousness is used as a kind of therapeutic tool that, in the end, amounts to another form of treatment not unlike the medical techniques it was meant to supplant. There is little explanation of the mind/body relation that sheds light on the actual problem and identifies the role of consciousness in such a way that underlying causes can be understood, not just applied in the form of treatments. To be complete, a true concept of mind/body unity requires a dynamic understanding of functioning that makes it possible to identify underlying causes, and in so doing, to prevent the problem as a positive process of growth. It requires that we be able to identify the role of consciousness in such a way that we can go beyond the need for treatment and educate the individual in the causes of illness and the possibilities of rising above it.

Understanding mind and body as a unified system (and how to raise the working of this system to a conscious level) is one of the key problems in the mind/body field, and yet it has hardly even begun to be articulated as a subject matter. Part of the reason for this omission is that the search for cures has obscured the need to understand underlying causes. When we suffer from a symptom, we are so oriented toward its removal that we hardly know how to look at the underlying functions from which it may stem. We are so intellectually dominated by the very notion of cure, of not having a problem, that we don't even have a concept of what function is. Broadly speaking, this idea has changed somewhat over the last several decades with the development of such fields as cognitive and developmental psychology. In the area concerning health, however, virtually no progress has been made toward developing a foundation of theory and practice. Mind/body concepts in medicine are so specific and symptom-oriented that the very development of the concept is concerned more with finding cures than with an appreciation of mind and body itself.

The articulation of mind/body unity, which is the subject of this book, demands that we identify the problem from a completely new perspective—that of the mind and body as a functioning system. Arriving at such a concept, as I will show, cannot be achieved simply by empirical testing of various techniques, and then building a theoretical concept on the technique. It must conceive of the mind and body as a functional system and demonstrate how to raise the working of this system to a conscious level. This process, as I intend to show in this book, is very different than simply demonstrating a link between mind and body, and it requires a far more subtle and sophisticated concept of mind and body than that conceived by clinical techniques now in use. The problem of consciousness, in this case, is not merely that of employing awareness for the purpose of producing therapeutic changes; it is the problem of becoming aware of and controlling one's own behavior from within.

The beginnings of this subject were first articulated not by medical science but through the work of F. Matthias Alexander. Alexander, an Australian actor performing around the turn of the century, discovered that in all movement there is a fundamental organizing principle that makes fluid and balanced action possible. Based on this discovery, he formulated a means by which harmful and stressful action could be kinesthetically perceived and prevented. These insights made it possible, for the first time, to describe in practical terms how the human organism works in movement, what is actually wrong when someone suffers from muscular tension, and how to consciously recognize and prevent harmful responses in oneself.

This approach to the problem of awareness in activity provides the beginnings of a unified theory of mind and body. Up until now, most mind/body theories have approached the mind/body problem by demonstrating the empirical effects of behavioral and relaxation techniques. When, however, the human organism is viewed in terms of how it functions in action, it becomes possible to address the more fundamental question of how to gain a conscious awareness and control of this system in activity.

That there is a need for such a concept may, to some, appear surprising, since the prevalent literature demonstrating the link between mind and body, and the power of consciousness to tap into this link, appears to provide precisely these elements. Yet the work that has been done in the field—useful as it is in the therapeutic domain—is far from complete in its conception of the relation of mind and body, or in bringing us forward to the full realization of the human potential that tapping this connection implies. In the field of psychology, for instance, it was long understood that a number of complaints that had previously been classified as medical no longer fit within that mold. In response to this recognition, there was a search for new techniques, such as hypnosis, to address these problems, and a conceptual framework was erected on the shaky foundation these techniques provided. But this was only the beginning of a fully elaborated field that, it later became clear, demanded a much more comprehensive understanding of subject matter as the basis for a true foundation of theory and practice.

We are in the same position with respect to the present investigation xvi ••• The Undivided Self

into the mind/body relation and the role of consciousness in controlling stress and tension. There has been an increasing recognition that problems that appear physical relate to a larger spectrum of elements. Many methods have borne this out in demonstrating the efficacy of new approaches, resulting in a new mind/body paradigm. This empirical construct creates the general impression that there is a static entity of the mind that somehow mysteriously affects the body, and that the only problem is how to harness this latent power. But it is not enough to develop methods for reversing the symptomatic manifestations of harmful conditions and then base a theory of mind and body on such empirical practices. It is necessary first to articulate the underlying function, or subject matter, of which they are a part, and to describe what is wrong as the basis for a fully elaborated theory of mind and body.

Taking this next step requires—as in the development of any emerging field—the discovery of new subject matter and a novel orientation to old subject matter. Even when psychology in its early stages understood that certain types of illness didn't belong to the usual class of medical problems, the methods employed to treat these symptoms were still largely framed from the point of view of the medical model that was itself inadequate to solve these problems. The mind/body field, at present, is at precisely this stage of development. It has recognized that particular classes of apparently medical problems have causes that are non-medical, but it still conceives the approach to these non-medical problems in largely therapeutic—and therefore medical—terms.

The treatment of symptoms, however, can be highly misleading as the basis for understanding the causes of problems, since what we think is wrong is often actually very different from what is actually wrong. Because we have conceived problems in terms of symptoms, we have looked with the same medical approach we are trying to break free of; even when we have recognized that particular kinds of symptoms do not yield to traditional treatment, we still rely on the old vocabulary for approaching these symptoms. In fact, the actual solution requires a new outlook and new knowledge; the very basis for the realization that these types of symptoms don't yield to traditional treatment is the corresponding fact that they emanate from undiscovered elements of human functioning. Addressing new problems requires the description of a new subject matter—in the present case, how the body functions in action as a unified system of mind and muscle.

If articulating a more comprehensive subject matter means a greater knowledge of what causes symptoms, it also implies a greater knowledge of the role of consciousness in addressing symptoms. At present, the mind/body field assigns to consciousness a central role in the treatment of illness, but this role is largely conceived in curative terms. In contrast, articulating the function of the living organism as a complex unified whole yields a far more sophisticated concept of consciousness, which is seen not simply as an antidote to symptoms but as a process of raising action and conduct to a conscious plane. If tension and stress are related to lifestyle and conduct, then consciousness cannot be applied purely in the context of clinical procedures. Conceiving the subject matter in this new way reflects the true role of consciousness—not as subservient to clinical results, but as the process of control itself.

The infancy of this field also implies a certain carelessness about practice. Few people would question the need, when undergoing surgery or facing a complex legal problem, for expert help. But because many mind/body procedures require little supervision, are practiced at home, and do not involve any overt danger, we often assume that such knowledge, like a home remedy, is universally available. As a result, people otherwise thoughtful and intelligent in addressing educational, medical, or legal questions accept the most thoughtless and questionable advice when it comes to health practices. When once we begin to articulate the true complexity of this field, however, we will no longer accept, from others or from ourselves, such careless and haphazard practice. As with any field, the subject of our own health and practical procedures relating to it are complex and varied, and must be based on sound practice and theory.

In this book, I want to look at mind and body not as the basis for applying a therapeutic method but as a complex functioning system and, by so doing, to begin to formulate the outlines of a theory about how this system works, what is wrong with it, and how to raise the working of this system to a conscious level. By identifying how particular symptoms can be traced to the wrong working of this system, it will then be possible to arrive at a greater understanding of the origin of these symptoms and what is involved in changing them.

The objection might be raised that the process proposed here is too elaborate. How, for instance, can we legitimately expect a person with a minor backache to analyze the entire spectrum of actions and reactions underlying the problem? We must keep in mind, however, that we are not always granted the luxury of deciding how much attention a problem requires to be solved. If my car breaks down, I do not complain to the car mechanic that I would prefer he only tune up my engine instead of repair it. Yet this is often exactly what we do in response to the problems addressed in this book: we decide one solution doesn't suit our pocketbook or calendar, and choose a more superficial one, even if it won't actually repair the problem. Even when what is required is short-term treatment, it is necessary to have a comprehensive understanding of the problem based on a solid foundation of theory and practice. If it is to be valid and useful, the immediate approach must first be seen in its larger context; then, at least, we can be reasonably certain that our approach will be educationally sound.

The need for immediate treatment, then, is a poor justification for not having a larger body of knowledge on which to base particular techniques. A practical exploration of the entire process of achieving conscious control is not for everyone, but the knowledge it represents is. As long as we continue to conceive this field in purely instrumental terms—as short-term techniques for personal growth or as a commodity for ailing clients rather than as a complex subject requiring serious exploration— we will continue to approach these problems in a haphazard way, without a real appreciation of what is involved, and we will deny ourselves the increased awareness and benefits in living that will naturally flow from this appreciation.

The Undivided Self

CHAPTER ONE

A Unified Model of Mind and Body

For many decades, two trends in psychology—nature and nurture—have competed to the point of exhaustion. Genetic theories, which lately have gained in repute, have demonstrated how profoundly we are influenced by our genetic heritage; Freud and Skinner, who epitomize the nurture theories, stress the susceptibility to environmental influences and the role of conditioning. Each tendency is presented as one of a two-sided debate; those who insist on the possibilities of free will lean toward the environmental side of the debate. Both points of view, however, share a common belief that we are influenced by factors beyond our control, and so have obscured a third possibility: the idea that, as human beings, we are capable of self-direction; that we can rise above genetic heritage and environmental influences by realizing our full capacities for conscious awareness and control in every phase of human life.

In this book I'd like to explore the possibility of raising the process of living to a conscious plane, not by introspection and analysis, but by understanding the mind and body as a functional system whose workings can be brought to a conscious level. We are so dominated by notions of cure that we think of mind and body as a kind of connection that can be exploited in order to produce therapeutic results, and are satisfied with techniques which produce results based on this link. But beyond these, and far more important, is the articulation of the mind and body as a system that must be brought to a conscious plane—a task that, because of the focus on cures, has yet to be undertaken. In attempting to do so, I am advancing a concept, not of sickness and how to cure it, but of the mind and body as a functioning system, and of how to raise the working of this system to a higher level of awareness in all aspects of living.

Prevailing Concepts of Mind and Body

According to the widely accepted view—to be opposed in this book—
mind and body communicate, or interact. It is now widely recognized
that problems that appear medical are often expressions of stress and emotional conflict and can be effectively treated through relaxation, meditation, and imagery. Out of this process has arisen the interactive concept
of mind and body. We no longer speak of mind and body as separate; it
is now well known that ideas, emotions, and beliefs influence physiology,
and that mind and body therefore communicate, or interact. The mind
is believed to hold latent powers capable of influencing the body through
techniques that tap into the power of consciousness and its potential to
influence physiology. In short, body and mind are communicating systems, and learning how they communicate is the key to improved health.

Among the many mind/body techniques now in use, we can distinguish at least three principal categories. The first regards bodily symptoms as expressions of emotional conflict, and thus conceives the
mind/body relation in terms of physical complaints that are either sym-
bolic expressions of mental events or a direct reaction to emotional states.
This view, epitomized in the work of Sigmund Freud, is perhaps the most
influential mind/body theory of this century. Asserting that physical complaints are in fact expressions of emotional conflict, psychoanalysis has
engendered the concept of psychosomatic illness, in which various physical problems, such as gastrointestinal disorders, tension, headaches, arthritis, and even cancer are linked to emotional states. Related to the
psychoanalytic and psychosomatic theories are the body-oriented psychotherapy theories of Reich, Lowen, and others. This body of work links
repressed emotions to bodily states, and thus conceives physical armoring and emotions "held" within the body as the key to various emotional
and physical ailments.

Body awareness techniques represent the second category of mind/body
theories. Because tension and stress manifest directly in the form of
physical states, such techniques attack the problem directly by employing awareness to reduce tension and strain, to produce greater relaxation
and physical mobility, and to improve mental attitude. Posture and mus-

cle tension are seen as the expression and basis of emotional attitudes, and are therefore the key to improved mental function and reduced stress.

The third category regards the body as subject to the influence of consciousness—mind over matter. It has long been known that mental attitude influences the patient's health. Belief in the doctor, faith in God, humor—all have been shown to produce measurable changes in immune function, muscle tone, heart rate, and the like. Based on these observed connections between mind and body, many techniques that employ mental imagery or alter mental attitude have been incorporated into traditional medicine. By empowering the individual to bring these factors under deliberate control, illness is viewed not as an irreversible fact of life but as an expression of lifestyle and, ultimately, of consciousness itself.

Rift Between Theory and Practice

Few of these approaches, however, fully realize in practice the objectives to which they aspire in theory. For example, a holistic treatment that is based on a theoretical concept of a mind/body unity, but which reduces the individual to a passive recipient of bodily treatments, is in fact dualistic, since it cannot truly conceive of a mental and physical whole or a process that can be understood and translated into educational growth. The same principle applies in the case of clinically-based mind/body techniques. Scientific and medical literature derive, in a very general sense, from a biological conception of the organism which, by definition, conceives mind and body as a whole. It does not follow, however, that methods that rely on such empirical literature are themselves holistic in the real sense of the word. Stress theory, for instance, conceives of the response to stress as a mental, physical, and emotional event; yet the methods proposed to treat stress are often crude forms of relaxation that completely fail to explain, not to mention address, the cause of the stress.

The same can be said for body-awareness techniques. These methods utilize awareness and relaxation to address patterns of tension but fail to recognize the fundamental link of movement with voluntary action, and so in the very process of asking the subject to be aware are invoking the habits that are themselves at the root of the problem. It is not sufficient to apply awareness to movement and then to frame a concept of mind/body unity based on this awareness; movement itself must first be conceived in terms of its subtle connection to mental function as the basis for arriving at a concept of awareness.

A number of current theories address the problem of mind/body unity by simply amalgamating both mental and somatic approaches, thus addressing the relation of mind and body by attacking the problem from both ends of the spectrum. But such approaches, however eclectic, completely fail to address the real problem of mind/body unity. It is easy to accept in practice that mind and body function as a whole; our entire biological and scientific conception rests on this assumption. But this does not mean that when we view muscular activity we have only to add the psychological ideas borrowed from introspective psychology, or utilize other "mentalistic" approaches, in order to arrive at a true concept of mind/body unity. Even the simplest action can be seen to be mental, not in the sense that it reflects something mental, but because it is part of a total pattern of response that is at once mental and physical, and of which psychological attributes are an integral part. Unless we understand the nature of this mental and physical pattern of response and articulate a psychology specifically oriented to this subject, our mind/body technique, however well-intentioned, will be spurious.

The mind-over-matter concept, which has lately replaced the psychosomatic model as the prevalent conception of mind/body unity, also betrays an inability, in practice, to bridge the gap between theory and practice. Because this model emphasizes the role of mental attitude in influencing the body, the mind is treated as a hidden entity with the power to influence the body in mysterious and unaccountable ways; the body, being capable of receiving mental influences at an unconscious level, is the visible entity that manifests the working of these unseen forces. The exact relation of these two entities, and the reason for the power of the mind over the body, are seen as inexplicable; the mystery is itself invoked as the basis for the connection. But why does consciousness influence the body, and why does a lack of consciousness lead to problems? A concept of consciousness must reflect not simply empirical benefits but must itself be based on an explanation of the underlying problem, so that we understand not simply how to address problems but how to identify the underlying cause of those problems and the process of growth that enables us to overcome them. While it appeals to our sense of the mind as an untapped source of power, the idea that the mind is a hidden entity that influences the body amounts to a conceptual rationale for our lack of understanding of the exact nature of this connection.

Although the various mind/body theories embrace an ideological concept of mind/body unity, each fails in practice to articulate a positive theory that utilizes this relationship except in a purely therapeutic sense. Ideologically, such conceptions appeal to a concept of unity and to the need for awareness and education; in practice, they treat a passive patient who, in spite of appeals to become more conscious, is not informed as to the causes of bodily stress or made more aware in any significant way.

Need for Positive Understanding and Theory

In contrast to these "interactionist" approaches, I take the view that mind and body must be described as a whole system, and that only by so doing is it possible to fully realize one's potential for conscious awareness in living. The popular conceptions that stress and tension are expressions of emotions, and that the mind influences the body and can therefore be harnessed as the basis for practicing a holistic way of life, have provided the public with new concepts of wholeness with which to replace the traditional medical conception of a passive patient. They cannot, however, substitute for the unified concept of mind and body that is necessary for becoming fully conscious of action and behavior as the basis for understanding the causes of tension and stress in living.

Such a conception, as opposed to purely clinical approaches, constitutes a true "holistic" perspective on health. We are accustomed, in diagnosing illness and in assessments of performance, to use empirical criteria as the basis for making judgments; empirical research is now widely used to document and scientifically validate various holistic techniques. Apart from the fact that almost any method produces measurable benefits (rendering empirical tests meaningless), there is the further objection that such empirical data, which can do little more than demonstrate the link between variables, fail utterly to provide a positive knowledge of functioning. This can come only from a clear articulation, in practice and theory, of the organism and its complexities as a functioning whole.

The Functional Unity of Mind and Body

According to the view that will be put forward here, muscular action is inseparable from mental activity, the two occurring as a complete pathway of activity. Accordingly, harmful physical states that are associated with stress cannot be adequately addressed through therapeutic techniques that treat the bodily condition separately from the mental "causes," but only by learning to gain a conscious awareness and control of this total pathway of activity. Because this activity is largely unconscious, it is necessary to raise it to a conscious level—a process that can be achieved only by raising self-awareness and conscious control.

The concept that mind and body work as a functional whole is far easier to accept in theory than in practice. In modern introspective psychology, behavior is so often seen as the result of underlying motives or emotions that we automatically assume that physical symptoms are the expression of emotions, not that action itself is the problem. But we are designed for behavior, for doing things; muscular action is not an expression of mental or emotional qualities but is continuous with the mind in action. This is true of mind as well: we so often think of "mind" in introspective and cognitive terms that we forget that it evolved, not as a factor that influences the body, or that makes meaning of the world, but as part of action and, therefore, survival. Understanding this is at the heart of a mind/body psychology that views mind and body as a functional whole.

One of the main difficulties that stand in the way of appreciating such a view, as we can see from the foregoing, is the instinctive need, demonstrated by all of us to some degree, to break the organism apart. We are increasingly aware of the tendency, in Western culture, to value mental and spiritual pursuits above physical and mundane ones. This prejudice taints our interest in the body in a general way, but it has another, more pernicious effect. Once we choose the body as crucial to our process of inquiry, we tend to see *only* the body; the more recent trends in introspective psychology have reinforced the tendency to assume that mental aspects of living are limited to internal states and beliefs with little connection with physiology. But physical tension is not merely physical, even when we understand this to include physiological and nervous processes; on the contrary, it involves a complex psychology that must be included in any physical description. It is necessary, then, as a first step, to acknowledge that the study of the body does not exclude the mind, that we must in fact imbue it with mind, and that only by doing so can we conceive the actual behaviors that are subconscious and need to be made conscious rather than appeal to cures and therapies. Patterns of bodily tension aren't an expression of behavior; they are part of the pattern of behavior itself.

A functional approach to psychology requires that we look at action—at functioning itself—as valuable. We are all aware that we separate mind and body, but one of the hidden effects of this separation is the devaluation of practice: we tend to value mental and spiritual activities over physical or mundane ones. This same bias applies to the study of psychology: we tend to value mentalistic aspects of functioning over mundane activity because what is mundane is physical. Yet if we are to gain a true understanding of this subject, we must learn to value the simple fact of our own activity as a thing worthy of study.

From the point of view of the observations made in this book, then, and the subject that is its focus—namely, the body—the present work is an attempt to do justice to a subject which often falls prey to a dualistic prejudice that sees the body as having little or no relation to the mind. But from the point of view of more mentalistic concepts in psychology, a true concept of mind-body unity has the opposite significance: by viewing mental function as intimately connected to the body, we are restoring the body to its rightful place—or at least one aspect of its rightful place—in the field of psychology.

A Unified Model of Mind and Body

The idea that mind and body are a unified whole is so basic to the modern scientific attitude that it is difficult for most of us to accept that in practice we subscribe largely to methods that classify problems as mental or physical and therefore separate body and mind. When faced with physical discomfort or tension, for instance, the idea is so deeply ingrained that we need to treat the body that we hardly question the validity of such an approach. Yet this approach flies in the face of actual knowledge of how the body works. In physiological texts, for instance, muscles are often depicted at the end of a nerve, showing how the muscle activity is the end-point of a total neuromuscular activity. This represents more accurately how the body actually functions than relaxation and psychosomatic models, which view tension as an expression of stress and emotions.

Even this simple physiological concept, however, hardly does justice to the complex reality of action. Only the most primitive actions begin with nerve impulses that exclude the brain; every time we think, move, or speak, the muscular actions that take place involve the higher cerebral functions as well.

This continuity of muscular action with volition can be represented thus:

mental activity ••••••••••• muscular tension ••••••••••• motor act

Notice in this diagram that muscular tension is no longer seen simply as a bodily condition that reflects mental states; mind and muscle form a continuous pathway, like different end-points on an electrical circuit. In this model, even the simplest physical action can be seen to be mental, not in the sense that it reflects mental stress, but because it is a total pattern of response that begins with mental activity and ends with a muscular act.

The concept that muscular tension is continuous with mental activity to produce motor acts is not new to biology and physiology, which of course view body and brain as one system, but it is new to the practical study of tension and stress. In the various techniques we normally employ to treat tension, we behave, for all intents and purposes, as if the bodily condition is not only separate from the functional workings of the brain, but as if tension is unrelated to activity—the very purpose for which it was designed. But harmful tensions are part of a total pathway of activity; it is this pathway, and not just the condition, that must be addressed.

This activity, however, is largely habitual, and this makes it difficult to control. Although we recognize that involuntary states of stress are largely instinctive, we normally assume that voluntary behavior, by definition, is within our control. But we must remember that even voluntary behavior is part of a total physiological process that is largely automatic and unconscious. We have the subjective feeling that we control most of our actions, but our ability to consciously choose actions represents only the fringe of a complex mental and physical process that goes on unconsciously for many hours each day and even, to some extent, during sleep.

Because of this, the problem of controlling muscle tension, or the condition of stress that accompanies it, is not nearly as simple as it might appear. Although it is possible to alter bodily conditions with relatively little effort, gaining awareness of behavior itself represents a much more fundamental educational problem that demands a larger understanding of functioning and behavior. If tension and stress are to be viewed, not simply as a bodily condition, but as part of a total pathway of voluntary behavior, they must be

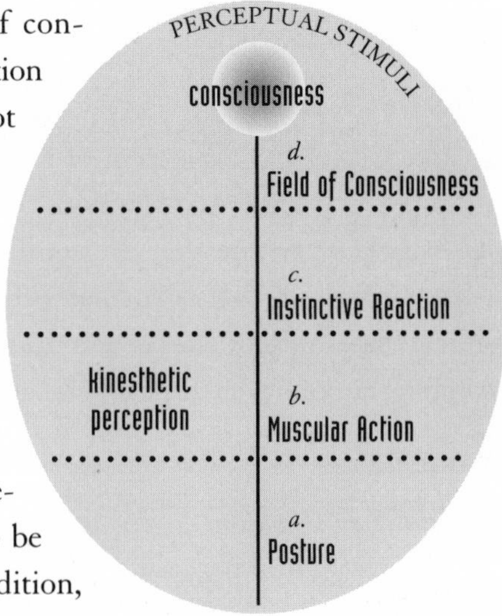

Diagram 1
Unified model of mind and body

placed within a larger functional context that must itself be understood in order to adequately identify the causes of tension and stress that occur in everyday life.

The diagram above illustrates some of the main components involved in understanding mind and body as a psychophysically functioning whole. It should be kept in mind that these various elements must be understood not in their usual context but as part of a functioning system. For example, instinct is used here, not in the context of a theory of personality, but in terms of involuntary responses which cause stress. Each of the components represented in the model is explained in more detail below.

a. Posture

Although muscles are connected with nervous activity to produce voluntary actions, they serve an even more basic function that must be taken into account in any awareness technique. In everything we do, muscles all over the body are coordinating to maintain balance and to bring about movement. Most of this activity is reflexive, or automatic; we become momentarily aware of specific muscles when we perform particular actions or experience muscle strain, but we are almost entirely unaware of the general working of this system. When, therefore, we experience strain in particular areas, we are unaware of the general condition of maladjustment and strain throughout the entire organism.

b. Muscular Activity

The second basic function of muscles is to produce movement. Even when we recognize that tensions are part of a larger pattern of strain, we fail to appreciate that the condition of tension is part of a harmful pattern of action that perpetuates the harmful condition. Muscular tension is therefore not simply a condition that can be treated but part of a complex neuromuscular pattern of activity that must be brought to awareness.

c. Instinctive Reaction

When faced with danger, animals and humans alike are designed to respond by fighting or fleeing, which is a protective response that ensures survival. This "fight-flight" response, which increases heart rate and other functions to permit quick and vigorous physical activity, is normal, but if it persists over time, stress-related diseases result. Many people are in a constant state of stress due to involuntary responses to stimuli that are perceived as dangerous.

d. Voluntary Action and the Field of Consciousness

Thinking appears to take place separately from bodily action, but in reality ideas are functionally linked with the muscular system and with motor activity, sometimes leading to overt action and sometimes not. Notice also that most of this mental activity is subconscious; only the fringes of this activity actually reaches consciousness. A heightened mental awareness must therefore be included in any mind/body technique for addressing bodily conditions of tension or stress.

e. Habitual Nature of Activity (not pictured)

Finally, notice in the diagram that muscular activity links not with the conscious part of the mind but with the much larger portion of mental activity that is subconscious. There are times when we are kinesthetically aware of muscular activity or momentarily aware of our mental experience; this portion of our mental life is conscious. But most of what happens, even in voluntary activity, takes place at a habitual, or subconscious, level. This explains why the pattern of activity is so difficult to change. Unless we become conscious of the pattern by raising the subconscious activity to the conscious level, patterns of tension and stress will remain for the most part outside our control.

Kinesthetic Awareness and Control

Such are the main elements that comprise a fuller conception of the actual living process of which tension and strain are merely symptoms. It should be clear, from observing this simplified model, that tension and stress involve a complex psychophysical process that must be understood in a comprehensive way if the cause of the problem is to be adequately addressed. When understood properly, stress and strain must be seen not simply as a bodily condition that requires treatment or specific control but as a complex behavior that demands an increasing awareness and control of the complex working of this entire system in action. When once we begin to gain a larger understanding of the elements involved in the problem, it also becomes clear that most people suffer from a maladjusted muscular system, faulty kinesthesia, and harmful patterns of tension. This activity is associated, in turn, with disturbance, loss of control, and increased stress in living. And if these problems are caused not simply by outside circumstances but by an imbalanced working of our own organism, then the challenge before us is not to reverse the ill effects of outside forces, but to identify the causes of the degeneration of our own species in our own activity.

Let us look now at the various steps involved in becoming conscious of this system in activity, based on an understanding of the organism as a functioning whole. We can lay out the following stages:

a. Bodily Coordination and Poise

b. Kinesthetic Awareness in Action

c. A Condition of Mental Alertness and Balance

d. Heightened Awareness and Conscious Control

a. Bodily Coordination and Poise

Although we are often aware of specific muscular tensions that cause pain, tension in fact occurs in the context of a complex muscular system that is engaged during waking activity to produce balance and support. This system works in a relatively unimpaired way in a young child, whose movement is fluid and balanced, and whose muscle tone is neither too high nor too low. With time, action becomes increasingly malcoordinated, resulting in physical collapse and strained, inefficient movement patterns. Through the process of kinesthetic re-education, the muscular system is restored to a naturally lengthened condition, returning a degree of poise and grace to the muscular system and reducing collapse and strain throughout the organism.

b. Kinesthetic Awareness in Action

Within the context of the larger system of postural muscles, specific muscles contract to produce movement, and in this sense are not simply part of the larger support system but part of an active system connected with the brain to produce activity. When this system is imbalanced, however, inappropriate muscular contractions interfere with the body's natural support, creating a condition of undue tension and collapse. When the muscular system is restored to a normal condition through a process of kinesthetic re-education, these habitual tensions can be perceived and prevented. This makes it possible to gain increasing awareness and control in simple actions that interfere with the natural fluidity and grace of the human body in action, reducing the condition of tension and strain.

c. Lowered Stress and Mental Calm

Because muscles operate continuously with the nervous system to produce action, muscle tension is part of a pattern of stressful response. In young children, muscle activity is balanced, and actions are therefore performed in a deliberate and calm manner. When muscular action is unbalanced, actions tend to be uncontrolled, and the corresponding mental state is distracted and preoccupied. The individual responds too quickly to even the simplest tasks, and becomes unbalanced and overwrought while performing simple actions or responding to everyday stimuli. This reactive tendency is also associated with a mentally preoccupied or worried attitude—that is, harmful emotional states that become chronic if persisted in over time. When the muscular system is balanced and harmful actions are kinesthetically perceived, the level of stress returns to normal, restoring a vital, calm condition free of nervous strain and worry. Harmful emotional states dissipate, mental alertness is restored, and there is a corresponding improvement in mental attitude.

d. Heightened Awareness and Conscious Control

Based on the three previous stages, it is possible to raise the normally habitual process of action to a conscious level. Muscular activity is normally controlled at a subconscious level and is therefore difficult to alter. When the muscular coordinations are so adjusted that muscle length is increased, it then becomes possible to kinesthetically identify the pattern of activity as it occurs, which means that the subconscious activity can now be perceived. This raises the habitual process of action to the conscious level, leading to a heightened state of awareness and control.

This awareness and control makes it possible not simply to reverse the ill effects of stress on the body but to prevent the underlying causes of tension and stress in action. By kinesthetically perceiving the muscular activity that occurs as part of the response, it is possible to gain control over activity that was previously subconscious:

kinesthetic re-education .... awareness of pathway of activity .... conscious control

Because stress is caused, not by outside stimuli, but by the organism's harmful responses to these stimuli, the key to the control of stress is the ability to identify how actions operate and to raise the process of action and reaction to a conscious level. This ability, in turn, is based on a unified concept of mind and body that views muscular action and mind as part of a functional system that can be brought under conscious control.

Standard of Psychophysical Health

The above elements provide the basis for a positive understanding of functioning and health that is grounded in a practical knowledge of how the organism functions as a unified system. The following concepts describe some of the basic areas that come within the scope of a unified approach to mind and body.

a. The Control of Tension and Stress

To be complete, a system for treating the symptoms of stress must offer a means of understanding the causes of stress in our own responses and behavior. This challenge cannot be adequately addressed based on a medical model, nor by employing mind/body techniques designed to alleviate symptoms, but only when the organism is understood as a unified system that functions in action. By gaining an awareness of the subconscious activity that underlies conditions of tension and stress, the process of reaction that causes the body to respond negatively to stimuli can be consciously perceived, raising these unconscious and harmful reactions to a conscious level. Such a conception makes it possible not only to recognize symptoms and how to relieve them, but to perceive the underlying process of activity that gives rise to these symptoms.

b. The Outlines of a New Field

The study of the organism as a functioning mental and physical system provides the foundation for a comprehensive theory of stress. Current stress techniques recognize the fundamental role of the mind in contributing to stress, but the effort to arrive at immediate cures has obscured the need for a positive understanding of how mind and body function and of how this system becomes misdirected and imbalanced. A true theory of stress must be grounded not in clinical practice but in a comprehensive understanding of mind and body as a functional system, and in the educational process by which the individual can gain an understanding and awareness of this system. These elements are not embraced by current medical or psychological techniques, but comprise a unique field of human psychology—the mind and body viewed as one functional system. Understanding this system provides the basis for a theory of stress that recognizes the possibility for education, and not treatment, as the basis for identifying the causes of stress.

c. Psychophysical Concept of Functioning

While educators recognize the need for a standard of physical fitness and mental health in the developing child, no such standard exists in the realm of psychophysical functioning. Various systems combine relaxation and stress-reduction systems with emotional work, and in so doing, hope to arrive at a comprehensive system for addressing mind and body. But a unified concept of mind and body describes a new aspect of functioning that is neither physical nor emotional health, nor an amalgamation of the two, but a new field entirely—the subject of the psychophysical working of the organism in activity. This concept makes it possible to establish a standard of *psychophysical*—as opposed to mental or physical—health in the adult and in the developing child. Such a psychophysical standard identifies not merely what is wrong in the child, nor simply a crude concept of fitness based on empirical tests, but a positive standard of functioning based on a practical knowledge of how the muscular system is coordinated in action and reaction, how this system becomes misdirected and imbalanced, and how to rectify this system through kinesthetic re-education and conscious growth. It offers a new standard of growth and development based on performance not in specific areas but in the use and functioning of the child's own organism.

d. Conscious Awareness and Control

Most important, a unified concept of mind and body makes it possible to understand the true potential for conscious development. Because the study of mind and body has been motivated largely by the need to find specific cures for stress-related disease, consciousness has been conceived largely as a therapeutic tool for producing immediate benefits in health; the true potential for conscious awareness and growth has been all but ignored. But problems that appear to be clinical in nature are in fact the result of our lack of knowledge about the human organism, its subconscious functioning, and the need for a more enlightened approach not just to health but to living itself. A unified approach to mind and body provides a practical means of raising the process of thought and action to a conscious level, making it possible thereby to prevent the onset of conditions leading to stress and to establish the foundations for a new approach to health based on conscious prevention and control. The concept of mind/body unity ultimately makes it possible to embark on a path of conscious development, leading to greater insight into the nature of one's functioning and, ultimately, to a heightened awareness and an awakened mind.

CHAPTER TWO

Origins of a New Field

The Behavioral Link Between Mind and Body

As I mentioned earlier, a great deal of literature on the subject of mind and body has proceeded on the assumption that, like other medical and clinical subjects, the mind and body can be studied empirically by employing methods for relieving conditions of stress and then observing the effects of these methods on muscle tension, emotional states, and the like. But if tension and states of stress are in fact not medical conditions but, as the new holistic point of view indicates, related to lifestyle, attitude, and emotions, then the solution of this subject demands not new methods but a knowledge of functioning and a consciousness of how we live that enable us to gain increased awareness in living. Such knowledge can be acquired only by gaining a conscious understanding of our own behavior—understanding ourselves from the inside, so to speak.

This is in fact how my own views on this subject originated: not from clinical or empirical studies on the subject, but from a practical effort to understand concrete problems from which I personally suffered. Such a point of view does not preclude clinical observation or empirical research, but the starting point and real source of knowledge in this field must by its very nature involve insight into the problem of behavior and consciousness of one's own actions. Accordingly, I will begin by outlining my own story, as it were, in order to provide the reader with the insights that led to the ideas set forth in this book.

I

My initial knowledge of this subject came about in the following way. Throughout my teenage years I engaged in a number of strenuous activities such as long-distance running, mountaineering, and other sports. By the time I entered college I was extremely fit by normal standards, but at the age of nineteen I pulled a back muscle and from that time on had chronic back pain that forced me to give up running and climbing, as well as piano and other activities that required sitting for long periods. In spite of my efforts to stretch, to perform relaxation exercises, yoga, and a number of other awareness techniques, my problem became not better but worse, and I became vaguely conscious of a loss of vitality as well as demoralized by my back problem, which by this time forced me to lie constantly on my back and to give up my normal lifestyle.

After experimenting with a number of methods for dealing with my problem, I came to the conclusion that all my efforts to physically correct the problem had failed because there was nothing wrong with me physically. I was convinced that if I were to solve my problem, I must treat not just the condition but must in some fundamental way identify how the tension was linked with the mind, and then learn to control the tension or become aware of it in some way. I began to search among the literature for methods that treated the mind and body as a whole, but was again disappointed. Although a number of authors appealed to a concept of mind/body unity, the actual procedures they used seemed either to treat the mind—which I didn't believe to be the source of my problem—or the body, which I did not believe in my case required therapeutic measures. I had also become skeptical of methods that were based on theoretical concepts of mind/body unity but which did not reflect in practice a true understanding of what this meant.

During this time I read the work of F. M. Alexander, an Australian actor at the turn of the century who had developed a system of awareness and control based on a concept of mind/body unity. Suffering from hoarseness during performance, Alexander had observed himself in front of a mirror and, by closely studying his movements, had discovered a pattern of physical tensions that were interfering with the normal functioning of his voice. Observing a tendency to tighten his neck and pull back his head when he recited or spoke, he found that the relationship of the head to the torso governed the body in movement, and that his pattern of tensions was interfering with his body's natural ability to function. This pattern of tension, however, was not simply physical. Alexander found that when he spoke the tension occurred in response to his desire, or wish, to speak; in this sense, the tension was part of a larger pattern of action and reaction that governed all forms of activity. When he was able to prevent this entire pattern from occurring, he reinstated the natural functioning of his muscular system and his voice returned to normal.

Based on this discovery Alexander developed a practical method for helping others to detect and prevent harmful patterns of tension and reaction which, he said, caused problems in functioning. By enabling the student to perceive the harmful pattern of activity, a teacher trained in his method could reinstate the proper relationship of the head and torso, resulting in an improved overall functioning. The process was not therapeutic but educational; the goal was for the student to become conscious of what he or she was doing, not be passively treated.

The educational emphasis of this process appealed to me, and I decided to go to a teacher for a demonstration lesson. Standing at my side, my teacher made some subtle alterations in the position of my head. She then asked me to sit down. As I did so, she pointed out that I made certain actions—for instance, arching my back slightly when I moved. When I asked her how she could see this without examining me, she said she was not assessing a bodily condition, but noticing small movements that were visually observable. These movements, however, weren't haphazard; they interfered with the natural length of the body that was organized by the head and spine. When I moved, I pulled back my head and shortened the spine, thereby interfering with the natural support of my muscles and ultimately causing my back to malfunction.

Adjusting my head and encouraging my neck muscles to assume a more normal length, my teacher then demonstrated what it was like to move with the head leading and the body lengthening in movement. I saw that, when I moved, I normally interfered with this length by pulling back the head and shortening in stature. If, instead, I "directed" the head up and the body to lengthen, I then began to experience movement as easy and effortless, giving me a feeling—one that often persisted for hours—of being lighter than air, of an internal system that was allowed, for the first time in years, to function as it was designed to function.

This capacity for lengthening in movement, Alexander had observed, was basic to all animal movement; it could be observed not only in cats and dogs, but in many children and in some adults who still moved with a fluid grace and poise. In the various sports I had played, however, I had developed the tendency to pull back my head and tighten in movement, which over time had interfered with this length, causing me to lose the natural effortlessness in movement I had enjoyed as a child. By consciously "directing" my head and torso, I could regain this natural ease and flexibility in movement, allowing the body to function more normally and to resume a more lengthened condition.

Even more importantly, this new head-torso relationship gave me an increased kinesthetic awareness that made it possible to detect what I was doing in action. When I pulled back my head, this action was so habitual that I had no awareness I was doing it. When the teacher adjusted the poise of my head, however, the increased length in the muscles of my neck made it possible to perceive that when I moved I then tightened in these muscles and pulled back my head. I could then begin to see that, in virtually all my actions and even in sitting, I tended to narrow and arch my back, as well as retract my head, which explained for the first time what I had been doing to cause my problem.

The concept that my back problem could be caused not by a harmful condition but by what I was doing in activity agreed with my experience; I had always intuitively known that my problem had been directly related to the way I had "used" myself. By being shown what I was doing, and by contrasting my harmful pattern of "use" with a more coordinated way of doing things, I could for the first time begin to prevent these harmful actions, and I began to experience periods of relief from my back trouble. I was convinced I was on the right track and wanted to know more about this subject, which I felt might hold the key to my back trouble and enable me once again to function normally. I decided to enter a teacher-training course in the Alexander Technique—a three-year course of study that involved, besides learning how to teach, intensive work on improving one's own standard of "use." This, I felt, would give me an opportunity not only to make a career out of a subject which had begun to fascinate me but, what was more important to me at the time, to have the opportunity to explore my own patterns of "use" and regain my own natural functioning.

II

After a course of lessons, I experienced a limited degree of relief from my back pain, but I was certainly not free of my problem. If, after a lesson, I had some feeling of lightness and reduced tension, I would lose the feeling within a matter of hours, if not minutes. The muscles of my back were still chronically tight, and I often found that my back pain persisted as before, particularly when I engaged in certain activities. I wondered whether in spite of my interest in my "use" and even commitment to it I would need further treatment or, worse, would never be able to overcome the tensions from which I suffered.

My subsequent experiences, however, were to prove how mistaken I was. I knew from my private lessons that when the teacher moved me from a sitting to a standing position I pulled back my head, which interfered with the relationship of my head and torso. I had repeatedly tried to alter the position of my head, thinking that if I could learn to move differently, I could solve the problem. With limited success, I felt that I was learning to move better and sometimes was able to re-create the feeling of length that I increasingly experienced in lessons.

What I didn't realize, however, was the extent to which this pattern of tightening had interfered with the natural functioning of my body. When I moved, I could now begin to see that I wasn't simply tightening my back or moving badly; the pattern of tightening was only part of a larger pattern of shortening and constriction in my torso, neck, and legs and was responsible for a deeper pattern of chronic tensions throughout my body. I wasn't just moving badly; I was literally collapsing my entire muscular system.

Furthermore, this pattern was not simply physical; it was a kind of response that would come into play, against my will, whenever I performed an action. When the teacher made adjustments, I found that, at the moment I was asked to move, I would grip and constrict, uncontrollably, throughout my body. Even when, after asking me to stop and not do anything, he would then move me again, I found that at the moment he did so I would become preoccupied with what he was about to do and stand automatically, without even realizing it was happening.

What I had thought was a back problem, then, was in fact far more

complex and extensive—a pattern of muscular response that was interfering with the normal working of my body. The body, I now learned,
had a system of internal postural support—or reflexes—that permit us
to move and support ourselves in whatever we do, without having to think
about what muscles we use. In animals, as well as in young children,
this system is normally working well; but with time, the pattern of tension in many adults interferes with this system to such an extent that it
literally cannot work properly, forcing the body into a compensatory
arrangement that makes various parts of the body become rigid and tense
and others collapsed and weakened, resulting in discomfort, pain, and
dysfunction. In my case, the muscles of my back had become so overworked that they literally could not function normally, operating for the
most part in a state of spasm and chronic tension.

What had appeared to be a condition of my back, then, had in fact
been symptomatic of a larger pattern of habits that had interfered with
my entire muscular system. My back pain did not indicate a problem simply with the lower back; it was part of larger pattern of tension that had
involved the whole body in a complex system of compensatory holdings
and tensions of which I had simply never been aware. By learning to
"direct" the head and back, and then to "inhibit" the instinctive or habitual desire to use my body in the way that had become customary, I
slowly learned to prevent this pattern of response, reinstating a more
normal condition of the entire muscular system and restoring the ease
and flexibility I had had, but lost, as a child.

Achieving an improved working of the postural system, however, made
it not easier but harder to maintain these changes in activity. If, after
bringing about an improved condition, my teacher then asked me to
perform a simple action without tightening, I didn't believe I could
move in any way except with the old tension; at the moment the teacher
would move me, I would instinctively react to what he was doing and
perform the action in the habitual way. Even in so simple an action as
sitting at a desk, I found that I had been shortening and using the system wrongly, without even realizing I was doing so; when I tried not to
shorten, the old tendency was so ingrained that it would come back,
within a few minutes, just by thinking about the familiar action.

The problem, I realized, was not simply that the body was itself malfunctioning, but that it operates, when we are actually using it, according to an instinctive process that simply isn't within our control. Like many animals, we have the power to decide what overall action we may or may not do, but once we decide to do that action, the entire nervous system is brought into play at a level that is almost entirely unconscious. It was not enough, then, to change the bodily condition; the process of action itself must be held in check, so as to create the possibility of learning a new response to the "stimulus" of doing something. Only by holding this instinctive process in abeyance, and focusing instead on the process, or means by which we do things, would it be possible to overcome this habitual pattern.

This process of focusing not on the "end" but on the means, demanded a level of discipline that had never before been required of me. This wasn't the kind of process that could be learned, as with many sports or even music, through repetition or effort; it required a mental attention and awareness that seemed all but impossible in actions that we normally do so habitually. There were times when, as I was about to get out of a chair or perform some other simple action, performing the action differently seemed all but impossible. At other times, I was sure I would be able to do the action in a new way, but found that at the moment I would actually begin to move, my old tendency to tighten and constrict had come into play, without my even realizing it. Slowly, however, I learned to focus more on myself, while postponing the "end" toward which I was working; the action would then take place with surprising ease and effortlessness.

When I was able in lessons to maintain the new pattern and to hold in check the instinctive one, I soon began to apply this principle to my own activities. When performing an action such as sitting down, the desire to sit (the "end") would instinctively bring into play the harmful pattern of tension and constriction. In order to counter this tendency, I would have to break the action down into component steps, in this way focusing away from the "end" of sitting down and shifting my attention instead to the process of "how" to perform the action. This ability to "think in activity," as John Dewey called it, required intense conscious discipline;

over and over I found that I became unconsciously preoccupied with the "end" and had failed to maintain focus on the process. Only by giving up concern with the end and focusing entirely on the means was I able to prevent my habitual response and the tensions that went with it.

Learning to perform actions consciously also made it easier to identify what I was doing in my daily activities to perpetuate these tensions. After repeatedly having the experience, in lessons, of performing a simple action such as inclining forward in a chair by shortening and tightening, I slowly became aware how much I must be doing this in all my activities. Because the act of writing at a desk or speaking on the phone was so ingrained and habitual, I had never before connected the harmful tendencies I had observed in lessons to the way in which I performed these everyday acts; but as I became consciously aware of my harmful pattern, I realized that, whenever I wrote at a desk, engaged in conversation, or walked down the street, I was indulging in these same habits, without ever having realized how destructive they really were.

At the heart of my difficulties, then, were my own actions, which I was now forced to examine, in virtually every facet of my life. The difficulty of replacing habit with conscious thought in the various activities of daily life was, I soon discovered, no easy task, but as I began to successfully apply what I learned to my various activities, my overall condition began to improve and, with it, my back. I discovered a new-found sense of awareness and control in all my activities and an increased sense of enjoyment in performing actions and learning new tasks. The focal point of this process—as many performers learn—was an ability to think in activity; in this case, though, the control was not specific to a particular skill but was applied to all forms of activity. By learning to stop and then redirect the body, I could perform actions in a new way; the result was a constant improvement in how I performed tasks and an increasing sense of enjoyment in doing things and learning skills that had become laborious and painful.

III

Based on what I had learned in the training course, I diligently employed the principles of the Alexander Technique in all my activities. But it was my later personal experience with this subject matter that led to my overcoming my problem and my subsequent attempt to describe the ideas set forth in this book. My intention, as I have stated in this book, is to define a new subject area—a reality which, as I hope has been made clear, was made possible through Alexander's discovery. A number of works describing Alexander's discovery have been written prior to my own, and so the experiences that led to my formulating my own ideas on the subject are in need of some account.

As I just mentioned, it is possible, through the help of a teacher, to restore an improved functioning of the body and to begin to perceive, with increasing clarity, the harmful pattern of tension that interferes with this normal functioning. After becoming versed in the procedures for achieving an improved working of my system, I became able, through my own application of these procedures, to bring about such improvements on my own, and after some time I was able to perform actions in a dramatically improved way—to sit more comfortably, to use my voice with less strain, and to perform other actions easily and skillfully. I began to understand not simply how to relax muscles but how to coordinate and control action more intelligently. I also gained the ability not simply to perform specific actions more skillfully but to become aware of the actual process by which I learned any skill.

This process, I had learned, was easily identifiable; the improved functioning was not the result of mechanically practicing movements or the haphazard result of becoming aware of whatever tensions I happened to notice. It came about as the direct result of a clearly conceived theory about how the body worked in movement, how to detect the harmful patterns that interfered with it, and how to replace these harmful patterns with intelligently thought-out actions that were consistent with the body's physiology. I had found the educational process I had been looking for.

But my problem was not entirely removed. Although I could, by this time, command an improved working of my body, I found that when I performed complex actions such as playing the piano or typing I was not able to maintain such improvements. After a period of even a few minutes, I could clearly detect a return to an overall condition of tension.

At first, I attributed this deterioration to the simple fact that my original chronic tensions had still not entirely disappeared; it seemed natural, therefore, that they would reappear when I performed the sorts of actions that had originally caused them. I became determined to continue making physical changes, hoping that through this process my condition would improve to such an extent that the chronic tensions would finally disappear.

But this did not occur, and I began to question what could be the cause of this persistent tension. Even after having a course of lessons and intensive training in the Technique for over a year, I was still subject to the same tensions that I had originally suffered from, albeit to a diminished degree. Could the method I was using be defective, or could my physical condition have deteriorated to the point that I could never expect to be entirely free of my original complaint? At first, I was inclined to answer both questions in the affirmative. My physical condition had been far from ideal; perhaps no method in the world could ever reverse such a problem.

Through the process of working on myself, however, I began to realize that there was a discrepancy in my reasoning. I had, by this time, become sufficiently capable of making changes in my physical condition so that within a matter of a few minutes I could bring about an improved condition, even if I had become considerably tense while typing or playing the piano. If I could so definitively reverse the harmful condition of tension, and if after playing the piano or typing at a keyboard the problem returned, I could then improve my condition again, where exactly was the problem? The piano was an inanimate object; clearly *it* could not cause me to become tense. And clearly the problem wasn't in my body, since I was able, each time it went wrong, to reinstate an improved condition. The problem, I concluded, mustn't be in me or in the piano; it must still be in what I was doing, if only I could find what that was.

So I began the process of sitting at the piano and, while playing a few notes, compared my initial improved physical condition to the harmful condition in which I later found myself, to see if I could identify what caused the deterioration and exactly when it occurred. At first, I could not detect the presence of any harmful tensions, or when they came about;

whatever activity was causing my problem was happening at a level of which I was unaware. However, after several more sessions sitting quietly at the piano and bringing about the improved condition, I began to perceive that at the moment I got the idea to play I tightened the muscles of my neck, back, and legs, and that this faint and almost undetectable pattern of activity began in direct response to my mental involvement in, or thought of, playing the piano. Whatever problem had existed physically, it was now clear, was perpetuated at a subconscious level by a mental and physical connection that, at its root, had nothing whatsoever to do with my body *per se,* but was fundamentally rooted in the habitual nature of my own voluntary action. At the heart of such a concept, I realized, was a link between ideas and a pattern of muscular activity that could only be described in unified terms; I could prevent the harmful pattern of physical activity only by becoming conscious of this link between mind and body.

In order to solve my problem, I realized that I would have to paradoxically learn to maintain the improved condition and play a note while somehow avoiding the idea of playing the piano. Through a process of sitting quietly, away from the piano, and consciously attending to my physical condition, I began to challenge myself to walk to the piano but to notice if at any point in the process I actually had the idea of playing. After some time, I found that if I sat quietly, the idea to rise and go to the piano would literally disappear from my mind; if I then decided to get up, I could detect when the mental involvement began. By recognizing this normally unconscious event and stopping each time it occurred, I found that I could make my way to the piano by degrees until I was sitting quietly at the piano, and that I could allow my hand to rise and strike a note without actually having the idea of playing. Through this process I was slowly able to replace my normal habitual process of playing with a conscious one. The final step was being able, while sitting at the piano, to play an entire piece in a state of heightened awareness in which I was able, by stopping and waiting, to replace my normally unconscious actions with actions consciously performed.

The key to the problem of conscious control, then, was being able to perceive the link between ideas and muscular actions that occurs below consciousness; this was the fundamental problem underlying my back problem and the cause of the stress I had experienced for many years. By learning to gain a coordinated and "directed" use of myself in activity, I was now able not only to perform physical actions in a new and effortless way, but to gain a conscious awareness and control over my actions, resulting in an increased control and balance in all my actions. Although I had progressed to this stage through the application of principles and pedagogical procedures, it was not possible, by mechanical means, to solve my problem. It was necessary, ultimately, to raise the process of activity to a conscious level by assuming full responsibility for the process and intelligently conceiving the problem.

Based on this experience, I came to the conclusion that in order to progress as a field this problem must be conceived, not in terms of a method, but in terms of the fundamental underlying problem—the problem of raising habitual action to a conscious level. My goal, accordingly, is to describe how the body works in action and what goes wrong with it, and to articulate the mental and physical connection that lies at the root of this physical problem. Such a problem requires a new vocabulary—a conception of how the mind and body function as a unified whole in activity.

•••

It should be clear from the previous discussion that the problem of mental and physical control which forms the subject of this book must be framed in the context not of clinical or therapeutic methods but on the basis of the individual's own conscious awareness and control. It is for this reason that I have given the preceding account. Apart from this brief discussion, however, I do not intend to resort to personal narrative in the remainder of this book. To begin with, personal testimonial is open to the objection that such experiences are subjective and therefore liable to self-deception. But there is a more serious reason for my choice. The problem of conscious control that is the focus of this book is fundamentally based on the underlying operation of habit, or instinct. Without articulating what this underlying process is, it is impossible for the claim of conscious control to have any meaning. Subjective narrative simply cannot fully do justice to the problem of describing this underlying function, which must be described in detail if the problem of conscious control is to be clearly articulated as a field.

For this reason, I have sought other means of communicating this insight—means that would allow both a clear description of the problem as well a lucid account of the various types of problems that fall within this category of human functioning. At first, no such means were available; insight into a problem does not by any means automatically confer verbal or conceptual clarity as to how to convey such insight. The existing literature on the subject—books about the Alexander Technique describing the concept of "use" and the method for improving it—do not provide much in the way of help, since they have largely focused on the physical benefits of practicing the method and downplayed the need for a serious treatment of the mental and behavioral aspect of the problem. Clinical studies and research methods tend to focus on the physical and symptomatic aspects of the problem, and so again do not provide a useful means of conveying the subtleties involved in action and how to become aware of such action. In short, neither of these mediums is appropriate to conveying the concept of mental and physical unity that is at the heart of this subject.

And yet the process of observation does in fact provide a means of communicating the subtle concepts of mind and body. In the course of my teaching—and I have seen hundreds of people over a period of seventeen years—I have had occasion to observe, in others, the same pattern of harmful muscular activity that I initially observed in myself, and I slowly began to perceive in these physical patterns of movement the same subtle mental processes I had observed in myself. Although we usually think of mental events as non-observable, they can in fact be clearly discerned under the right circumstances. If I could describe these circumstances accurately, they would provide an ideal means of communicating the mind/body concept I was trying to convey.

I should add that, to a large extent, such a methodology does limit the scope of what can be presented, since once I did find the means of external observation that is the basis for communicating the ideas set forth in these pages, I was prevented from being able to present more anatomical and practical information. This method also tends to favor the viewpoint that the problem is behavioral, and so precludes the possibilities of describing clinical and pedagogical problems. Communicating this subject, however, has proven to be even more difficult than coming to a practical understanding of the problem, and it has been necessary to sacrifice fuller elaboration on certain topics, which I hope to redress in the future, to the essential topic of mind and body which is the focus of this book.

Accordingly, I will take, as the object of study, a more or less fictional student, whom I will observe in various activities. Beginning with the study of physical movement as a point of departure, I will then progress to the relation of physical movement to mental function and finally to the problem of conscious control. Before entering into the topic of mind and body, however, I will review the work of F.M. Alexander, who originated this field of inquiry.

Development of a Technique

F. Matthias Alexander (1869-1955) was an Australian actor who specialized in giving one-man recitals. A demanding performance schedule took a toll on his voice, and he began to experience recurring bouts of hoarseness that threatened to ruin his career. Forced to solve his vocal problem or else give up the stage, he made a series of detailed observations of his vocal use to see if he could find the cause of his problem.

In *The Use of the Self* (1932), Alexander gives a detailed account of these observations and how he finally solved his problem. During normal speech, he could detect nothing unusual in his manner of speaking, but once he began to recite, he saw that he tended to "pull back the head, depress the larynx and suck in breath through the mouth in such a way as to produce a gasping sound" (1932:9). Believing that these tendencies constituted a misuse of the voice, Alexander began to experiment with ways of preventing this pattern, during which he realized that the specific tensions of the head and neck were in fact part of a larger pattern of tension that involved "undue tension" throughout the organism.

At first, Alexander reports, there seemed to be no way to prevent this harmful pattern of tension, but through experimentation he found that although he could not directly prevent the tendency to suck in breath or to depress the larynx, if he could prevent the pulling back of the head the other two tendencies were reduced. He also noted that if he combined this forward movement of the head with a lengthening in stature, this overall adjustment was associated with an improvement in the condition of his throat. Based on this experience, Alexander arrived at the initial conclusion that lengthening his stature by putting his head forward and up constituted the "primary control" of his use in all his activities, and that interfering with this pattern had been the cause of his vocal and respiratory difficulties.

These initial changes, however, did not entirely solve his problem. Attempting to maintain these improved conditions while reciting, he found that in fact he was unable to do so. Suspecting that he might not be doing what he thought he was doing, he then realized that although he thought he had been continuing to put the head up and to lengthen in stature while reciting, in fact at the critical moment he was putting the head back—"startling proof," he wrote, "that I was doing the opposite of what I believed I was doing and of what I had decided I ought to do" (15). The reason for this deception, Alexander observed, was that in everything he did he used himself habitually "in the way that felt natural." This feeling, however, was not actually reliable, and because of this he simply did not have the control over the actions that he thought he had:

> I was indeed suffering from a delusion that is practically universal, the delusion that because we are able to do what we "will to do" in acts that are habitual and involve familiar sensory experiences, we shall be equally successful in doing what we "will to do" in acts which are contrary to our habits and therefore involve sensory experiences that are unfamiliar (16).

The assumption, then, that the pattern of misuse could be changed by voluntary effort was a wrong one, and Alexander was forced to re-evaluate his efforts thus far. He knew that he had been doing something to interfere with his voice, and he had discovered, as he wrote, what that "something" was. But whenever he tried to prevent this pattern, his efforts invariably failed. One of the reasons, he observed, was that his wrong manner of speaking—the pattern of interference in the head, neck, and torso—was intimately bound up with the incorrect working of other parts of the body, and this formed a complex pattern of interference that could not be prevented simply by altering the use of specific parts:

> Observation in the mirror shewed [sic] me that when I was standing to recite I was using these other parts in certain wrong ways which synchronized with my wrong way of using my head and neck, larynx, vocal and breathing organs, and which involved a condition of undue muscle tension throughout my organism (17).

This pattern of tension was further complicated, Alexander recalled, by his training as an actor. When he had studied dramatic expression and elocution, he had been told to "take hold of the floor with his feet," and his misguided efforts to carry out this instruction had further disturbed his overall equilibrium and use. These tendencies had all combined to form a deeply ingrained complex of habits, and they were brought into play any time he attempted to recite or, for that matter, perform any action:

> I then realized that this was the use which I habitually brought into play for all my activities, that it was what I may call the "habitual use" of myself, and that my desire to recite, like any other stimulus to activity, would inevitably cause this habitual wrong use to come into play and dominate any attempt I might be making to employ a better use of myself in reciting" (19).

At the heart of the difficulty, Alexander observed, was that this "instinctive misdirection" came into play as the result of a decision to use his voice. "Over and over again," he writes, "I had the experience that immediately the stimulus to speak came to me, I invariably responded by doing something according to my old habitual use associated with the act of speaking" (27).

In order to address the problem, Alexander adopted the following plan.

First, he must "inhibit" the immediate response to the stimulus to speak. Second, he must project the directions for the primary control and continue to project them until ready to employ them for the act of speaking. Finally, he must continue to do so and then, at the "critical moment," reconsider whether to go on to achieve his end, do something entirely different, or do nothing at all. By following this plan, Alexander said, he was finally able to maintain the new use while reciting—a process, he said, that not only alleviated the harmful condition of his voice, but also had a marked effect on his functioning in general.

Based on this experience, Alexander began to teach a "New Method of Respiratory and Vocal Re-Education" that was founded not on the performance of specific exercises but on preventing harmful habits of breathing. Most breathing and vocal techniques, he noted, were based on the assumption that the student needed to perform particular actions and ignored the presence of pre-existing harmful habits that interfered with the normal working of the respiratory system. In particular, Alexander warned against the popular conception of "gasping," or "sniffing" in air, and the raising of the chest and other unnatural movements that accompanied the student's effort to get enough breath. Instead, the student must have the "correct mental attitude," as well as the proper "pose of the body" and "poise of the chest." This way, Alexander argued, respiration can take place naturally, lending a natural strength and expressiveness to the voice. "I do not claim to have discovered any new method of breathing," he wrote, "but to understand the only true one—Nature's" (1995:39).

At first, Alexander focused on difficulties with breathing and vocalization, but with time he began to apply his technique to a broader range of problems such as scoliosis, consumption, back trouble, muscular aches, general loss of vitality, and various nervous problems. Analyzing harmful patterns of activity that interfered with the muscular system, Alexander focused on reinstating the normal role of head and torso in organizing movement.

Improving the student's general coordination, however, was virtually impossible when based purely on verbal instruction. Through experimentation, Alexander developed a means of conveying kinesthetic experience to the student by the direct use of his hands. By learning to alter the dynamic balance of the head in relation to the torso and employing other similar procedures, Alexander developed a practical technique for redistributing muscle tone and reinstating the proper conditions of coordination. In this way, he could demonstrate the lengthening response to a student in a short time. Even more important, the changes in muscle tension provided "a background of feeling tone" against which the tension pattern could then be perceived, making it possible for the student to gain control over habits that had previously gone unnoticed.

In 1904 Alexander decided to go to London, encouraged especially by a prominent surgeon who felt that only there would Alexander's work become recognized. With letters of introduction from doctors and theater people, Alexander set up a private practice in London and taught there until 1914. Although he continued to work with actors, he began to extend the influence of his work by publishing several pamphlets on respiratory re-education, in which he first introduces the concept of "conscious control," which is achieved through "re-education." In these pamphlets, Alexander also challenged medical practice on the grounds that its diagnosis of illness was incomplete because it ignored how a person's way of doing things affected his or her functioning.

This connection, Alexander wrote, demonstrated a fundamental principle in health and functioning—namely, that "an unsatisfactory manner of use, by interfering with general functioning, constitutes a predisposing cause of disorder and disease..." (1932:92–3). The whole problem, Alexander argued, was that many organic and so-called medical problems had their root in the wrong "use" of the self. Furthermore, when a medical problem was treated in the conventional way—that is, by treating the specific symptom—Alexander found that it left these predisposing causes untouched. For this reason, he felt that:

> no diagnosis of a case can be said to be complete, unless the
> medical adviser gives consideration to the influence exerted upon
> the patient not only by the immediate cause of the trouble (say,
> a germ invader), but also by the interference with functioning
> which is always associated with habitual wrong use of the
> mechanisms and helps to lower the patient's resistance to the
> point where the germ invader gets its opportunity (1932:94).

Between 1910 and 1941 Alexander wrote four books in which he advanced a theory about conscious control based on a unified view of the organism. The "mental" and "physical," he argued, were only convenient ways of describing an inseparable whole. "If any reader doubts this," he later wrote,

I would ask him if he can furnish any proof that the process involved in the act, say, of lifting an arm, or of walking, talking, going to sleep, starting out to learn something, thinking out a problem, making a decision, giving or withholding consent to a request or wish, or of satisfying a need or sudden impulse, is purely 'mental' or purely 'physical'" (1932:5).

"When once it is recognized," he argued, "that every act is a reaction to a stimulus received through the sensory mechanisms, no act can be described as wholly 'mental' or wholly 'physical.' The most that can be said is that in some acts the 'mental' side predominates and in others the 'physical'" (1932:43). He maintained that in a civilized state man's instincts could not be relied upon, and that humankind was tending to degenerate more and more. If he was going to survive, he would have to learn to rely on conscious control. He also argued against methods that, characterizing a problem as mental or physical, recommended various exercises or methods. Instead, he said, man would have to be treated as a whole, and would need to learn to bring his own reactions under conscious control.

During the early years of his work, Alexander did not have the benefit of a physiological explanation of the response that he had learned to produce. But during his lifetime he came into contact with the work of two scientists—Sir Charles Sherrington and Rudolph Magnus—who threw light on his discovery. Sherrington, a prominent English neurologist, had done extensive study of the various reflexes, or nervous pathways, that account for the complex actions of animals. By "decerebrating" animals (disconnecting parts of their brains), he had demonstrated the existence of involuntary reflexes that were responsible for movement and posture. Magnus, a student of Sherrington's, had taken a particular interest in the postural reflexes, and expanded the work of Sherrington by identifying and describing in detail the many reflexes governing balance and movement. For instance, when raised above the floor and dropped on its back, a cat will attain the four-footed posture by involuntarily righting itself

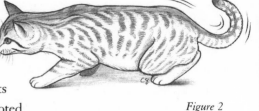

Figure 2
Attitudinal reflexes in cat

in relation to the gravitational field; this Magnus termed the "righting reflex" (1924:244). When stalking a mouse, however, the cat will automatically assume a posture that will enable it to run or jump in order to catch its prey; this he called an "attitudinal reflex" (1925:345). (See Figure 2.)

The most striking feature in Magnus's observations, however, was that these movements appeared to be organized—as Alexander had claimed—through the relation of the head to the body. When assuming a position, Magnus wrote, "the mechanism as a whole acts in such a way that the head leads and the body follows" (1926:536). (See Figure 3.) The head/neck reflexes were thus a "central mechanism in orienting the animal to his environment" (Jones 1997:47). Since this discovery seemed to correspond to Alexander's discovery of the key role of the head and neck in organizing human response, supporters of Alexander's work credited Alexander with having anticipated in his practical observations on himself and his students the laboratory discoveries of Magnus. Adapting Magnus's concept of a "central mechanism" ("Zentralapparat"), Alexander used the term "primary control" to describe the key role of the head in organizing movement and posture. The movements he had initially observed in himself—the pulling back and down of his head, the lifting of his chest, the narrowing of the back and tension in the legs—constituted an interference with this mechanism. This interference had increased with time and especially as a result of wrong habits that he had acquired from voice teachers and in performance. When he had been able to prevent this interference and maintain the proper lengthening during speech, this reinstated the proper working of the "primary control," which was associated with an improved overall functioning of his voice.

The Method of Kinesthetic Re-Education

By making adjustments in the relationship of the head to the torso, an experienced teacher of the Alexander Technique can produce the lengthening response of the "primary control" in a subject in a few moments. When this relationship is established, one experiences a "kinesthetic effect of lightness." This experience of lengthening, or lightness, which is the hallmark of the Alexander Technique, is easily capable of being demonstrated. As Frank Pierce Jones, a scientist who conducted research on Alexander's work, writes:

> *Applying a light pressure with his hands, the demonstrator changes the balance (or poise) of the subject's head in such a way that the muscles in the nape of the neck lengthen, allowing the head to rotate slightly forward as it moves up from the shoulders.... The demonstrator then helps the subject to continue the changed relation between the head and trunk during a few everyday movements like walking, sitting down and standing up, or raising his arms. In the process the subject's body can be felt by the demonstrator to lengthen and become lighter. Subjects regularly report that the movements are easier and smoother and that they feel lighter and taller while they are doing them (1997:5).*

This kinesthetic effect, Jones said, can be demonstrated for almost any activity, and "the sensory effect of lightness that accompanies the guided movements persists often for hours and sometimes for days, affecting the patterns of all subsequent movements" (1997:7).

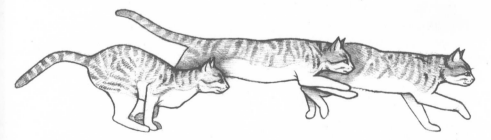

Figure 3
Cat leaping, showing how the head leads and the body follows

The reason for this effect, Jones says, is the changed relationship of head to torso, which elicits a muscular response to counter the effect of gravity—what he called an "anti-gravity mechanism." Living in a field of gravity, a human being must be able to counter, or neutralize, the effects of gravity: that is the function of postural muscles. Because the head/torso relationship is crucial to the working of this system, reorganizing this relationship lengthens and stimulates habitually contracted muscles in the neck and spine, with the result that upright posture is experienced again as effortless, and the body regains a sense of lightness and buoyancy.

The anti-gravity mechanism, according to Jones, has several components. The head is balanced on top of the spine in such a way that its weight tends to drop forward. When the head is poised properly on top of the spine and is not being pulled back, this tends to lengthen the spine. It also tends to exert a stretch on the muscles of the neck and back, stimulating stretch reflexes that in turn support the entire structure. Upright posture is then achieved with a minimum of effort, the various parts of the skeletal and muscular system working in a balanced way. (See Figures 4a and 4b.) In this way, the entire structure responds to the downward force of gravity by actually maintaining an upward force, so that "a movement against gravity is facilitated by gravity itself" (Jones 1997:143).

The civilized conditions of daily life, however, tend to interfere with

HEAD BALANCE AND UPRIGHT POSTURE

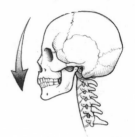

Figure 4a
Head balance

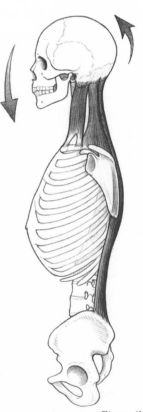

Figure 4b
Head balance and
extensors of neck and back

this mechanism in humans, causing postural malformation and conditions of tension. By making adjustments, a skilled teacher is able to restore the proper working of the "primary control," bringing about a condition of "true relaxation." This restores the student's faulty "kinesthesia" and improves the ability to discriminate between necessary and excess tension in the various acts of daily life.

After the student becomes familiar with this improved condition, he is then taught to observe the way in which he performs actions on his own, and to apply the procedures for an improved functioning of the "primary control" to daily tasks. By "inhibiting" his immediate and unthinking responses to situations that interfere with the fluid action of the body, the student learns to replace his habitual actions with consciously directed activity. In so doing, he not only restores his natural poise but also acquires the means of accomplishing daily tasks in a new and more intelligently worked out way.

Inhibition is a key concept in Alexander's work. Corrective and therapeutic techniques attempt to rectify harmful states by teaching the patient to do something to counteract the existing condition. Alexander insisted on the need not to correct what is wrong but, as a first step, to identify the harmful action and prevent it. The only way to achieve this was by stopping the harmful habits at their source—in other words, by refusing to act—a process that, borrowing from neurophysiology, Alexander called "inhibition."

Inhibition, as Alexander conceived it, is not a negative but a positive process. In the usual Freudian sense, inhibition implies repression of impulses. In neurophysiology, however, the term has a more positive connotation. As Sherrington, the neurophysiologist, wrote:

> It has been remarked that Life's aim is an act not a thought.
> Today the dictum must be modified to admit that, often, to
> refrain from an act is no less an act than to commit one, because
> inhibition is co-equally with excitation a nervous activity"
> (Sherrington, 1937).

This is the sense in which Alexander used the word. By preventing the immediate and unthinking response to a stimulus, inhibition thus makes it possible not simply to refrain from action but to choose how to respond constructively to the situation.

Inhibition, however, is not sufficient to prevent the harmful pattern of use, since the old harmful response must be replaced by a new one. When, therefore, the student thinks of sitting, he must stop and mentally project new directions to the "primary control" ("neck to be free, head to go forward and up, back to lengthen and widen"). The student is to project these directions for the head and torso simultaneously and sequentially, continuing to give directions for the first part while giving directions for the second part, so that each direction becomes part of a total pattern. When performed skillfully, these mental directions begin to elicit a natural, reflexive response in the body and, as this happens, they become a learned process that maintains itself unconsciously.

The ability to replace blind doing with thoughtful direction is, however, not easy for most students. When asked, for instance, not to pull back the head but instead to "direct" it forward and up, most students, thinking they have to "do" something, will try to perform the action by actually moving or positioning the head. This behavior betrays the underlying belief that, when we must change something, the only way is to *do* something to correct it—that "the defective action on the part of the pupil can be put right by 'doing something else.'" (Alexander 1946:128). "Forward and up" of the head, however, refers not to a posture or position, but to a dynamic balance of the head that results from an absence of interference in the muscles of the neck that pull the head back. And the only way to achieve this dynamic balance is by being aware without actually trying to "do" anything.

The problem is that when we conceive of muscle activity, or the ability to influence muscle tone, we normally think in terms of actions such as raising the arm, which produces a definite contraction, or tensing, of the muscle. Being asked to simply "think" of allowing the head to go forward and up seems, in contrast, vague and intangible. And yet it is possible to affect muscle tension just as concretely by using our awareness as by actively doing something. Consider, for instance, the insight that has been provided by biofeedback research. John Basmajian, one of the early researchers of biofeedback, attached very fine electrodes to muscle fibers, amplified the responses, and hooked the electrodes up to an oscilloscope in order to visually display the nerve impulses on a screen. He found that when subjects could observe the oscilloscope and therefore had feedback about activity in their muscles, they could learn to consciously control them with only a few minutes of practice. After a few more minutes some subjects were able to gain this control without the benefit of the oscilloscope, relying only on their own kinesthetic feedback.

This ability to consciously "direct" muscle activity graphically demonstrates the power of thought to make concrete changes in muscles. If the head is pulled back and the muscles at the nape of the neck are tightened, then by mentally directing the head forward and up it is possible to release the tension in the nape of the neck and restore the natural poise of the head, with no effort whatsoever. In the biofeedback studies done by Basmagian, subjects learned to control specific parts of specific muscles. But by directing the head in relation to the torso, this conscious power can be utilized not to control specific muscle fibers but to control the overall balance of tension governed by the head and torso. If the body is collapsed, "directing" the head in this way "energizes" the muscular system by restoring length; if muscles are overly contracted, directing the head releases excess tension. In this way, conscious "direction" results in a tangible change in muscle tone throughout the body, restoring natural muscle length by removing the unnecessary tension that has interfered with the primary control. And this result is eventually achieved, without the teacher's help, simply by "thinking."

The ability to direct the muscular system without the aid of a teacher, however, represents an advanced stage of the process. Since the typical student is in a state of tension and collapse, he cannot at first be relied upon to bring about the required changes on his own because his own sensory feedback is unreliable; it is up the teacher to give to the student the new experience of a correct overall working of the primary control by making the necessary adjustments. This process, however, is not simple, and often requires a good deal of time and skill on the part of the teacher. The teacher must diagnose the particular defects present and deal with various complicating factors. He must at times, depending on the sort of defects that prevent the correct working of the body, manually support parts of the body. If, for instance, the student tends to collapse or slump, he must put the student in "positions of mechanical advantage"—positions that bring about a natural lengthening of the musculature and proper reflex activity. He must also know how to release unnecessary tensions and to eradicate defects in the physique that interfere with the muscular reflexes. At the same time, the teacher must help the student be aware of these changes so that he can eventually make them for himself. This improvement in coordination tends over time to relieve the student of unnecessary tensions and to improve his overall functioning, and gains him a greater awareness and control over action.

CHAPTER THREE

The Body and Its Inherent Design

The Pattern of Tension

We observed from the outset that the mind/body field is rife with methods that offer a means for effecting particular changes in tension, stress, and bodily states, but that these methods fail to articulate a positive theory about what is causing the problem and why. This is because, in most cases, the various competing methods and theories are based almost invariably on therapeutic effects such as lowering blood pressure, relaxing muscles, and the like, and not on a substantive understanding of how we function and what is wrong with our functioning.

Perhaps this oversight is due to the fact that the cause of the problems these methods are meant to address is often unrelated to the symptoms themselves. Certain illnesses present symptoms that directly lead to their cause; in contrast, however, back trouble usually stems from activities that have no apparent connection to the symptom. In the same way that clinical depression may manifest behaviorally in the form of unproductive work, and yet emanate from childhood, problems of tension and stress often present no apparent link with their causes.

Some symptoms, however, do in fact present clues to their origins, and this begins to reveal a new subject area whose study, in the reverse direction, uncovers the origins of the symptom. In the previous account of F. M. Alexander's work, for instance, it was clear that what appeared to be a problem with his vocal tract was in fact the result of years of misuse of the voice due to faulty training and harmful vocal habits. Through patient analysis of his vocal habits, Alexander was led to a clear understanding of what he was doing to cause the vocal problem, and to a comprehension of the true origin of his symptoms. By thus tracing the problem in the original direction—not backwards from the symptom to the cause, but from the original faulty use to the symptom—it is possible to frame the outline of a new field of inquiry that will lead to a clear understanding of the cause of certain types of stress and tension.

The same principle holds equally true of the mind/body relationship, which is the focus of the present study. Various practices demonstrate or utilize the connection between mind and body, but because they neglect to trace the causes of the problems being treated, they are equally ineffective in making this connection meaningful. By tracing the original pattern of activity that leads to the symptom, however, the true relation of mind and body can be observed, demonstrated, and rested on a solid foundation of theory and practice. The study of this subject, then, must begin with an observation of the organism in activity; this, as I explained in the introduction, must come not from an outlining of methods to be followed that offer cures or effects, but must flow from a patient description and understanding, in actual practice, of the organism and how it works in action, as well as an identification of how it is being interfered with and how this interference leads to specific symptoms. It must define mental and physical forces not simply in terms of clinical practice but in substantive terms that increase our understanding of human psychology. And it must offer a means of raising the awareness of the individual concerned, so that he or she is able to gain a greater control over harmful activity through awareness and understanding.

Observing what we're doing while we're doing it, however, is not easy. We all experience tensions in the course of an average day; after having worked for several hours at a desk, we can often identify particular areas that are tense or strained. It is easy to assume, however, that we know what muscles are being overused, when in fact the act of working at a desk involves an extremely complex neuromuscular activity throughout the entire body. It is impossible to tell, based on subjective impressions, what we are doing with this entire system.

If, however, we observe others perform various activities, we can observe differences in levels of effort and strain. Observe an elderly person get up from a chair, for instance, and then compare this movement to that of a child. The child will perform the movement easily and effortlessly; in contrast, the elderly person will make a labored movement, sometimes even using his arms for support. One person walks and moves lightly and gracefully; another trudges along heavily, straining awkwardly to make even the simplest movement.

These observations, however, are haphazard, and in fact tension in movement follows a systematic pattern that can be observed. If you ask someone to rise from a sitting position, you will notice that at the point of beginning the movement he will slightly retract the head by tightening the neck muscles. This neck-muscle tension will be accompanied by tension through the shoulders, back, and legs, which will increase as the person rises onto his feet.

Understanding this pattern of tension provides the key to altering it. If you slightly adjust the balance of the head so that the muscles at the back of neck lengthen, this will exert a stretch on the muscles of the back, whose tone will improve; at the same time, the torso will tend to lengthen. This lengthening in the muscles of the neck and back will increase sensitivity to changes in the level of tension. When the person again prepares to move, he will then be able to perceive the increase of tension and to maintain the natural length and support of the torso during movement. When he then stands up, there will be a change in the overall quality of the movement, which will involve less muscular effort and a reduction of bodily strain.

I should point out that performing this procedure is by no means easy and should not be attempted by an untrained individual. If the head is adjusted in such a way that the neck muscles are overly stretched, the result is that the neck muscles, instead of releasing, will tighten. The procedure I am referring to, then, requires the skills of a teacher specifically trained in the ability to make changes in the muscular system and experienced in how this system is designed to work in movement.

When once we identify this pattern of tension in movement, it can be observed easily in a number of activities. Take, for example, the act of bending to pick up something. Most people, when bending over, will retract the head forcibly as if to counterbalance the forward movement of the torso. The result is a strained and awkward movement, performed with a great deal of muscular effort. If, in contrast, the neck-muscle tension is again detected and prevented, it becomes possible to lower the body by simply bending at the knees, without a marked increase of muscular effort in the neck and back.

This pattern of tension is particularly evident in those who are performing desk work. If, for example, you observe someone writing at a desk, you'll notice how his sitting posture will seem to conform to the activity: he will curl his body around the pen and twist his head and neck to one side while slumping downwards toward the desk. This postural pattern, however, is only the visible manifestation of an underlying pattern of tension. If a skilled teacher again produces a stretch in the muscles of the neck by adjusting the head and lengthening the spine and muscles of the back, the underlying tensions that cause the harmful slump become evident. The moment the writer again puts pen to paper, he will begin the action by tensing the muscles of the neck, retracting the head and raising the shoulders, and the body will be forcibly shortened into a slump by muscular tension in the neck and shoulders, the entire postural change resulting from an increase in tension. Again, the writing "slump" appears to be bad posture, but when you actually watch it in action, it is clear that it is, in fact, a pattern of tension that, like the act of standing, begins with tensing of the muscles at the back of the neck and throughout the body.

The awkward and strained movements we can observe in others correspond, then, to a concrete pattern of muscular activity, and understanding this pattern makes it possible to change it. When we begin a movement, there is an increase in neck-muscle tension and a retraction of the head. By adjusting the head and releasing the muscles in the neck, the tension can be perceived and prevented, reducing the tension and producing a more efficient movement.

But why does movement begin with an increase of tension in the neck, and why is the relationship of the head and torso crucial in preventing this pattern of tension? When the writer tenses the muscles of the neck, shoulders, and back and contracts the body into a slump, there is an overall increase in muscle tension. By altering the poise of the head in relation to the torso, it is possible to prevent this increase in muscular tension. But the writer's slump involves more than muscle tension. When the writer goes into his slump, the body as a whole is dragged downward toward the chair, and this downward pressure actually interferes with his sitting balance, causing him to fall back against the chair or, conversely, to resist this collapse by arching the back and sitting up straight. When, in contrast, the adjustment of the head sets up a stretch in the muscles of the neck and back, the body tends to lengthen and without any apparent effort regains its natural support against gravity.

The reason for this response is that the body is designed to support itself against gravity, and the pattern of tension interfered with this response. When we sit or stand, we don't maintain an erect posture as if we're pillars that have rigid structural support. Our muscular system maintains this upright posture by acting, in conjunction with the skeleton, to set up a support structure so that in writing—as in any other activity—the body will maintain its balance against the pull of gravity. This makes it possible to achieve an erect posture with a minimum of tension, encouraging an elasticity and balanced muscle tone throughout the body.

This overall support represents a different function of muscle than we're accustomed to. Normally, we think of muscles in terms of specific movements, such as raising the arm at the elbow. When we voluntarily decide to make such a movement, the biceps muscle contracts and the arm flexes at the elbow. In other words, the muscle has a specific function that corresponds to the specific action we decided to make. But the first, and primary, function of muscle is to support the entire body against gravity—in other words, to maintain the body's general support so that it is in position to perform whatever specific movements may be necessary.

This explains why the head and torso work together the way they do. Because the main structure of support for the body is the spine, it is the dynamic relationship of the head to the spine that maintains the musculature in the state of stretch that properly activates this support system to work. When this system operates properly, the muscles of the neck and back are maintained in a state of elastic tone that supports the structure; this inherent design in the system enables the body to maintain its basic support in all activities with a minimum of effort and strain. If there are unnecessary tensions, they will tend to interfere with this general system; but in any case, all specific actions take place within the context of the dynamic relationship of muscular tone organized by the head and torso that constitutes general postural support.

In the writer's case, though, this overall lengthening response had been interfered with, and it resulted in an overall loss of support against gravity. Because he has no consciousness, or knowledge, of this muscular system, the writer is aware only of specific tensions, and will therefore try in a haphazard way to relax his muscles or alter his sitting posture. But in fact his tension follows a particular pattern that corresponds to the working of the overall postural system, which he has interfered with by tensing and shortening muscles that need to remain lengthened. When that muscular length is restored to normal, he is then able to regain his overall poise and balanced support, as well as a more balanced distribution of muscle tone.

The tension we experience in performing simple movements or in working at a desk is not then a vague expression of stresses that somehow manifest in our bodies. When we feel "tense," we typically experience this tension during work and so attribute it to an outside "cause" that has to be removed in order for us to feel relaxed again. But the muscular system is an identifiable structure in the body that, for better or worse, serves its general and specific functions as part of movement and action, and the "tension" we experience indicates a disturbance in the body's system of muscular support that can be identified as a change, or alteration, in the poise of the head in relation to the torso, and a corresponding increase in tension throughout the body. Because we experience not the general pattern of tension but localized discomfort, which is often difficult to alleviate, we assume muscular tension is random and uncontrollable. But muscular tension follows a predictable and observable course, and when we understand the main elements that organize it, its origins can be identified and removed.

Observing this pattern provides a criterion for understanding muscle tension and strain that arise during activity. When the writer suffers from muscular tension, he knows something is wrong because he is physically uncomfortable. But because his judgment is based on subjective criteria— namely, his discomfort—he has no means of determining what is actually wrong, or whether he is himself causing the problem. But muscles serve a particular function in relation to the parts of the body to which they connect. If the head is retracted during writing, then the muscles along the neck and back—which connect directly and indirectly to the head—cannot possibly release, whatever efforts he may make to relax them. In order to release the back muscles, it is necessary to alter not the muscles alone but the relationship of the parts to which the muscles connect.

Muscular tension, then, is not a purely subjective condition somehow mysteriously linked with something internally "wrong" with the back or other parts of the body; nor can it be reduced to a diagnosis of specific muscles that have become shortened and need to be relaxed. In performing any movement, or when we are at rest, the muscles in the back are maintained at their proper length by the relationship of the body parts to which they connect. If we have a problem, it isn't just "happening" to muscles: it means there is a disturbance in the balance of the head and its relationship to the torso as it relates to movement and support. In other words, muscular tension does not exist independently of how the body works in movement, but is intimately related to it, and being able to observe movement is the key to a practical understanding of how muscles work. When observed in this context, we can identify how muscles have become tightened and why, and how to restore muscles to a more lengthened state. This length is organized primarily by the relationship of the head and torso, and when we understand this design, we can begin to make sense of tension as a recognizable pattern of interference with the human support system, and therefore as a subject area requiring detailed study and knowledge.

The Specific Complaint: The Case of Richard

Having taken a general view of the harmful pattern of tension that occurs during activity, I would like to turn to a more detailed case study, which will lead, in later chapters, to the problem of the relation of mind and body that is our focus. As I mentioned earlier, one of the difficulties in writing about this subject is to find a way of communicating subtle concepts in a way that is clear and concrete. In the course of my own professional experience, however, I have seen many people who exhibit the qualities I intend to convey; accordingly I will describe a typical case, from my own teaching experience, of someone (we'll call him Richard) who suffers from lower back pain; he exhibits a harmful manner of using himself, which appears to be at the root of this symptom. Using this case study as a point of departure, I will then describe various aspects of this problem, progressing in subsequent chapters from the apparent physical symptom to the larger mental and physical whole of which it is a part.

We observed a moment ago that, when someone suffers from a particular symptom, this does not mean that he is aware of the pattern of tension that may be giving rise to this symptom. Tension in a specific region of the body is invariably part of a total interference in the natural lengthening response of the body, and this larger interference of the head and torso is almost entirely unconscious. As I said earlier, observing the muscular pattern of head and torso provides a general standard by which we can assess specific conditions of tension and what might be causing them.

But in most cases, altering the relationship of the head and torso doesn't make it possible to entirely remove this tension. In the case of Richard, who as I said suffers from lower back pain, it is clear that the tension in his back, which can be easily felt, is associated with an arching of the back, as well as with a retraction of the head and a stiffening in the legs. It therefore seems likely that reducing the overall pattern of tension may eliminate this strain altogether. But in spite of whatever changes are made in the superficial pattern of movement, there is still an underlying level of effort and strain in his system. When observed closely, for instance, his rib cage is held in a kind of rigid pose; his chest is raised; his back is arched. In short, the tension pattern is associated with an underlying pattern of shortening and postural rigidity that has become ingrained from years of misuse, and the body has to be readjusted constantly to overcome a chronic tendency to strain and shorten throughout the entire system.

At first, it appears that by making specific adjustments in Richard's rib cage or shoulders, it may be possible to eliminate these postural rigidities and imbalances; but because the specific conditions are part of a total pattern of imbalanced action, direct attempts at specific adjustments do little to alter the entire imbalance and strain in activity. Even after making various adjustments, and again demonstrating to Richard how to move in a way which allows his entire system to remain lengthened, he continues to tighten and constrict, perpetuating the harmful condition of tension and postural rigidity.

As the stretch and elasticity of the muscles of the neck and back improve, however, there is a reduction of strain and shortening in the system, and the postural distortions are reduced, allowing the body to be naturally restored to a condition of greater ease and freedom and to regain its full stature. At first, these changes produce merely a sensation of lightness and support. But as the muscles change, there is an actual lengthening through the back and legs, a filling out of the back, and a general sense of increased mobility and reduced effort in action. Areas of the musculature that were tense begin to spontaneously release, allowing the system to become springier and lighter in response to gravity.

Even more significant, this overall change is associated with an improved working of the back. We saw, for instance, that the back was shortened, or hollowed, and concluded that this shortening needed to be reduced in order to allow the back muscles to function normally. But the shortening in the back was in fact directly related to the rigidity in the torso, which fixed the rib cage in such a position that the back became arched as a result. It was also related to tension in the legs, which caused the pelvis to tilt and further hollowed the back. As the system responds as a whole, this produces an alteration in muscle tone in these related parts, which in turn reduces the shortening in the back muscles and makes it possible for the back to function normally.

These postural changes demonstrate, at a deeper level, why Richard suffered from back trouble, and what changes need to take place in order to improve his condition. In the last chapter we saw that there was a pattern of tension that directly related to the body's natural support against gravity, and that reducing this tension allowed this system to function with less effort and strain. But it is possible to fully lengthen against gravity only when each of the parts of the system that comprises the whole is balanced posturally, and works in coordination with other, related, parts. In Richard's case, the tension pattern had created postural imbalances and distortions that constituted an interference with this system, and the back problem was symptomatic of this larger pattern of strain and maladjustment. When the interferences with the postural system were removed, this allowed the torso to regain its natural support, and the strain and interference were removed. So although it appears that the back problem is a specific condition, it is in fact symptomatic of the overall maladjustment in the working of this total mechanism. When the entire system is restored to its normal balance, the condition associated with that imbalance is indirectly eradicated.

This change highlights a crucial element in the problem of tension and strain. We saw, first, that there is a pattern of tension that interferes with the body's natural postural support against gravity. This gave us a general criterion for assessing how the body works and what we do to interfere with it. But the body's ability to lengthen against gravity involves a complex system of support that requires for its proper functioning the coordinated working of the various parts of the muscular system; the tension pattern had interfered with this coordinated working. Because the postural system cannot work efficiently, the various parts of this system are forced to work in a strained and harmful way. When the interferences with this mechanism are removed, however, the system can naturally right itself, or respond against gravity, and the various parts—including the back—can assume their proper functions, without direct treatment.

The interference in the overall working of the muscular system is therefore a critical factor in understanding—at least at the physical level—Richard's problem. Attempts to correct the body, whether by exercise, stretching, or specific treatment, may make a momentary change or give some immediate relief, but the body has an inherent design—a postural mechanism whose function is to provide support against gravity—and it must work in a balanced way. If the tension has interfered with that mechanism, then the true problem isn't to treat the specific condition, or even to lengthen muscles, but to restore the proper working of the mechanism that the tension has interfered with. When this happens, the various parts of the system can resume their normal function in the context of the whole. The problem is addressed not directly but indirectly, by restoring the natural working of this total system.

To give another example, take the case of someone with stiffened neck muscles. Anyone suffering from such a condition is likely to assume that because no other part of the body appears to be in difficulty, the problem is localized and must be treated specifically by relaxing the neck muscles. But close observation will reveal that the back, legs, and shoulders are also overworking and chronically tight, causing the body to twist to one side and to shorten in stature. Efforts at changing the specific condition of the neck may yield some slight or momentary benefit, but because the entire system is out of balance, it is impossible for the neck muscles to assume their proper tone so long as the total condition remains unchanged.

When the entire system is readjusted and restored to its natural lengthened state, however, this length evokes the natural response of the body against gravity, with the result that the various parts assume their normal function within the whole, and the specific problem is eradicated indirectly. Again, what appears to be a specific problem is in fact symptomatic of a total pattern of interference in the working of the entire muscular system. When this system is allowed to work properly, the overworked neck muscles no longer have to perform functions for which they are not designed, and are able to naturally relax and to regain their normal flexibility.

Understanding the total working of the muscular system, then, is a key element in solving particular kinds of tension-related problems, and shifts the focus away from specific treatment of symptoms. When we suffer from a symptom, the presence of pain indicates that something is the matter; we are so ingrained with this concept that even if we recognize that the symptom is connected with our activity and muscular use, we still insist that something is specifically wrong and requires treatment. This attitude is further reinforced by anatomical conceptions that, to even the least medically inclined, dominate our views about muscles and how they work. Even when, as in traditional anatomy, we have a concept of postural muscles that function as groups and that serve larger and more general purposes than specific muscles, we cling to the view that these specific muscles or structures are in need of treatment.

As we've seen in the foregoing examples, however, what appears to be a specific problem is often in fact symptomatic of the disorganization of an entire system that has been compromised by our own imbalanced muscular activity and use. This general organizing principle explains why a particular problem such as neck tension often does not require corrective or manipulative treatment. Even when we recognize that tense neck muscles are in fact part of a larger pattern of strain and maladjustment, it is still tempting to think that there is in fact something wrong—if not with the neck itself, then with muscle groups or structures. But specific symptoms will often disappear when the interference with this larger system is removed. The challenge therefore becomes not to correct what is specifically wrong, but to restore the normal working of this system.

The Mechanism of Poise

We began by asking whether it was possible to address the problem of tension not simply by treating it therapeutically but by understanding more fully what was causing it. By visually observing the pattern of tension, we have now progressed several steps in the direction of our goal. We first saw that tension, far from being a vague manifestation in the body, can be concretely observed in the form of a disturbance of the head-torso relationship. This relationship is a basic organizing principle in movement, and the pattern of tension has interfered with this system, leading to various compensatory adjustments and dysfunction. But why is the system organized in this way, and what causes it to become impaired, as it has in the case of Richard?

If you observe a child in movement, you can see a balanced, graceful action of all parts, and a fluid, solid movement of the whole. Even when performing complex actions with the arms raised, or sitting for long periods without back support, young children appear to exert little effort and experience no strain or discomfort.

This capacity for grace and effortless in movement can be observed even more easily in animals. It is rare to see a cat move awkwardly or strain in any way; virtually every movement it makes is a picture of poise and fluidity. Even when a cat makes a strenuous movement, such as leaping onto a tabletop high over its head, its body doesn't tense but actually lengthens as it springs from the ground. When at rest or in motion, its breathing seems fluid and effortless. After periods of strenuous activity, it seems to return to a restful state with little difficulty, and when it is sedentary, it seems never to lose its flexibility or ability for vigorous muscular exertion.

We saw earlier the governing principle in such movement. The head and trunk are organized in such a way that, in all movement, the spine can serve as a supporting structure for movement. In animals, this structure is horizontal, and the lengthening of the trunk, accordingly, takes place in a horizontal plane; in humans, the trunk lengthens vertically. In both cases, however, the structure is designed to support us against gravity with a minimum of effort, and the main organizing factor is the relationship of the head to the trunk.

The human erect posture, however, is much more delicate and unstable than the four-footed stance of animals, which explains, at least in part, why tension so easily develops in humans. Even so basic an action as sitting can, within a few moments, become disturbed if a child is asked, at too young an age, to control the movements of a pen while sitting at a desk. As soon as the child begins to write, he or she will begin to contort the body in order to control the movements of the pen, resulting in a slumped and tense overall posture. Such a momentary disturbance of the basic upright posture is easily rectified, but if it continues day after day, the muscles that maintain upright posture will eventually be taken out of gear, and the body will have to compensate in order to fulfill the basic imperative of maintaining upright balance, resulting in a chronically tense condition and postural distortion.

Like any dynamic system, then, the postural mechanism that supports us against gravity tends to work less and less efficiently the more we misuse it. With age, the condition of muscles, bones, and ligaments deteriorates until, with repeated and persistent harmful "use," muscles become chronically tight, and the overall condition of the body conforms to the distortion imposed upon it. However, if length is restored to the system, the innate working of the postural system is reinstated, postural rigidities and tension are reduced, and the body is again free to work as nature intended it—as an innate system that works reflexively, or automatically, to support us against gravity.

This reflexive component of the postural system is critical to fully understanding how the postural system works and how to reinstate it when it has become impaired. Usually we conceive of automatic systems as being inside the body, such as the heart, which automatically pumps blood throughout the body, or the digestive system, which chemically processes food without our even realizing it is happening. The postural system is "automatic" as well, though in a different way. Consider, for instance, what would happen if, when you rose from a chair, you had to figure out exactly which muscles to bring into play, and how much to contract each one. From an evolutionary point of view, it makes sense that we are capable of deciding which actions we will take. But precisely because we need to act efficiently, the body automatically takes care of the general support and muscular action that make specific voluntary action possible, so that, when we have chosen an action, we don't have to figure out exactly what muscles to use and in exactly what way.

The postural muscles, then, comprise a reflex system that is automatically stimulated into activity in everything we do, and precisely because these reflexes work in such a constant way, we are not aware of their active nature. Take as an example the act of sitting upright. It may appear that when an infant learns to sit up, the only "action" taking place is the act of balancing him or herself upright. The child's trunk seems to be solid and stable, and upright posture seems to be possible mainly because the baby can prevent itself from falling over. In other words, the body appears to be a kind of pillar, able to maintain erect posture because it appears to be structurally rigid. In fact, though, the baby's head and torso and legs are stabilized and supported by an ongoing and complex muscular activity, and it is precisely because that activity is so efficient and so constant that it is not apparent.

When this system is working incorrectly, though, and we then re-evoke the response against gravity, the truly active and spontaneous nature of this system is revealed. Without any apparent effort, the body regains its natural spring-like action against gravity; it actually feels as though standing and sitting require less effort than usual, and there is an increase in overall stature, a natural opening of the rib cage and chest, and an increased freedom of rib movements that allow breathing to take place more fully—all as a natural response that requires no effort or conscious decision. This upward spring-like force is so palpable that it is possible to evoke an improved pattern of movement in a subject without any intervention or conscious effort on his part. We saw earlier, for instance, how the average person has to brace throughout the entire body to rise from a sitting position, the entire pattern of tension constituting a shortening and tensing action. When the anti-gravity reflex is working, however, it is possible to stand the person onto his feet, with little increase in effort, simply by inclining his torso forward over his feet: as the center of gravity passes over the feet and the legs extend, the body effortlessly rises due to the support provided by the natural spring-like action of the torso. As long as the head is not retracted and altered in its balance–an action that interferes with the reflex support of the entire system—it is possible to perform this movement quite effortlessly.

Even more important, this reflexive response has an integrating influence on the different parts of the body. In Richard's case, we saw that the back had become hollowed, and that this condition was associated with strain in the muscles of the lower back and legs, which caused the pelvis to tilt and contributed to the hollowing of the back. When the entire system is restored to a condition of balance, however, there is not only a decrease in overall tension, but the parts quite literally "integrate" with each other, the pelvis dropping to work in a more fluid way with the legs, and the back regaining an overall stability and fullness as the ribs are restored to their natural flexibility—the entire process occurring as part of the natural coordination of the various parts of the body as they are designed to work in movement.

Corresponding, then, to the principle that the body as a whole must be taken into account in order to understand the correct working of specific parts is the principle that the system is self-organizing, or designed inherently to work as a coordinated whole. The muscular system has an innate design, an ability to reflexively organize itself in relation to gravity, and no specific treatment or healing process can match this inherent capacity of the body to organize and balance itself in preparation for movement. Strengthening one muscle group, or treating a specific region of discomfort, may sometimes provide immediate relief, but one has only to consider the general condition out of which such problems emerge to realize that an appreciation of the total system and how it works is an absolute necessity if the problem is to be addressed in a comprehensive way. The key to Richard's back problem is not to treat or reduce tension *per se,* but to restore the natural working of the overall system that permits the back muscles, as a key component of this interdependent system, to assume their proper role.

But perceiving the postural mechanism, and what may be wrong with it, is by no means easy. If you flex the arm at the elbow, you are likely to be aware precisely of the activity of muscles involved most directly in that action—in this case, the tensing of the biceps. Most exercise techniques, in fact, focus precisely on the capacity to tense particular muscles as the basis for developing and strengthening the body. But even so simple an action as flexing the arm is deceptively complex. In order to perform such a movement, the entire shoulder must be stabilized by muscles that connect to the back and torso, which are in turn connected with muscles that support the body in standing or sitting. In other words, specific muscles such as the biceps always work in the context of the total supporting network of postural support.

As I said earlier, then, the postural system is, first and foremost, a background system, and this explains why we are not normally aware of it. In contrast to the action of specific muscles, the ability of the body to support against gravity represents a general and nonspecific function of muscle, and precisely because this function is so basic, we are not aware of its operation. Our voluntary actions and intentions may dominate our conception of what we are doing with our muscles, but these specific actions reflect only a fraction of what is actually happening, at any given moment, in our muscular system.

This explains why Richard's problem—and its relation to the total system—is so difficult to identify. If, while performing simple actions, he has developed a tendency to tense and arch the back, as well as the neck and legs and other related parts, he is no more likely to be aware of this generally harmful condition than if his back were working normally. To a skilled observer, these defects may be easily observed. But because the working of the postural mechanism cannot be subjectively perceived, Richard has no way of assessing whether, when he experiences pain, the overall muscular system is in a harmful state. He is likely to assume that the problem is a specific "condition" that is limited to the area where he experiences the pain, and that his problem therefore requires direct treatment or corrective measures. Only when he is educated in the working of this system can he begin to understand that his problem is not localized but is symptomatic of an imbalance in the entire system. When this system is restored, specific maladjustments tend to correct themselves, and this natural righting process brings about a normal working and functioning of the specific muscles and parts that depend upon this total system.

CHAPTER FOUR

Ideo-Motor Action

The Subconscious Aspect of Use

At the beginning of this work, I set forth to examine the origins of the problem of everyday stress and tension, and we have now made some definite progress in this direction. In performing the actions of daily activities, there is a harmful pattern of tension that interferes with the natural working of the muscular system. This muscular system is organized by the relationship of the head and torso, and preventing the interference in this relationship makes it possible to reestablish a normal level of tension and muscle tone.

It is important to reiterate that the tensions we have been observing are significant not simply because their treatment offers a cure, or because relieving them provides immediate benefits, but because they represent an interference with an innate system. Understanding this system provides the basis for seeing how the muscular system works, and for identifying what is wrong with it. In the many works on the subject of tension, rarely is there any full and informed discussion of how the body works; usually there is a kind of myopia on the subject, even in the field of medicine, as if tension can be eliminated simply by performing a simple exercise or reducing stress. Perhaps for this very reason, the study of the body affords, for the patient student, a tremendously fruitful and rewarding field for study. Perhaps this is also the reason for the many relaxation methods that immerse the practitioner in an endless process of attempting to release specific tensions without any real understanding of what causes the tension to begin with.

But the study of the muscular system in movement is only the beginning of the problem, not the end. I said at the outset that the study of the body in activity in fact involves the mind and body as a total system, and that the key to understanding this field is to appreciate the combined operation of these mental and physical factors; this is the subject I want to now turn to.

We observed earlier that the average person, when engaging in a simple physical act such as rising from a sitting position, tenses the neck, back, and legs, interfering with the natural length of the body. By reorganizing the balance of the head and trunk, we saw how this tension could be reduced, allowing a natural system to operate, which in turn ensured an improved functioning of the entire system. By thus viewing this pattern and its improvement, we formed a basic picture of how the body ought to work. In Richard's case, we saw that although he suffered from back trouble, immediate treatment of his back played little part in the process of helping to restore his physical system. Observation of his particular pattern of activity revealed that he was misusing the various related parts of the muscular system; accordingly, the basic goal was to observe the elements that contributed to the wrong working of this pattern and to restore it as a whole. Having this picture in mind begins to give us a kind of goal to which we must strive when in the process of helping someone who suffers from a specific complaint of this kind.

But exactly how is this to be accomplished? Because Richard has a particularly pronounced tendency to constrict the muscles of his back whenever he walks, speaks, or performs other simple movements, it is necessary not only to restore the lengthened quality to the torso, which will allow the back to regain its normal tone, but also to prevent the tension that occurs as part of the pattern of activity. By adjusting the head and torso so that the back muscles are less constricted, he then has only to maintain this new condition while moving. In practice, however, it is not so easy for him to do this. Once he actually moves, he tends to contract his musculature, collapse, and shorten his body, in order to accomplish the action he is being asked to perform. In other words, he associates the activity of moving with the shortening response, so much so that as long as he needs to do any action, he feels he must unnecessarily tighten his muscles to do it.

Another possibility is to move Richard vicariously. Since the shortening of the neck and back muscles occurs when he deliberately moves, then one need only perform the movement mechanically for him, and it should be possible to stand him onto his feet without the usual pattern of tensions coming into play. But this approach is equally ineffective. If, for instance, I explain to him that I would like him to stand but that instead of moving himself I would like him to allow me to move him, and I then begin to move his body forward over his feet, at the moment I do so, he will anticipate my action and tense his body, in quite the same way as before, and stand on his feet, oblivious of my request that he not move at all. Even when I reiterate my point that I don't want him to do anything, and that I want him to stay where he is while I again attempt to move him myself, he again will tense in readiness to make the action. At the moment I begin to move him, he will jump into action, as before, tightening throughout his body and standing onto his feet.

This uncovers a new and unexpected problem in the study of the harmful pattern of tension and use. We have already observed how Richard performs actions harmfully, and so are not surprised that the tension pattern recurs when we move him. But whereas in other cases Richard has intended to make an action, this time it was not clear whether he was supposed to make the movement or not, and yet the action occurred automatically once I moved him, making him repeat the tensions even against his own will. Why, exactly, does he anticipate my action, and why does he do so even though I have asked him not to move and he has himself tried not to?

At first, the answer seems to be that he is simply reacting to the situation out of tension or apprehension. Being asked to perform a movement in a new way introduces an element of anxiety. Also, he is being asked to stand on his feet, and he could fall if he allowed himself to come forward in the chair and did nothing at all to assist. But this doesn't entirely answer the question. When I continue to perform the action, he continues to make the response, even when he is considerably more relaxed with the situation. Also, if I choose a simpler action—say, raising his arm—the same response occurs. Let's say that I tell Richard I would like to raise his arm and that I want him to do nothing, so that if I were to lift his arm and drop it, it would fall by his side. Again, at the moment I raise his arm, he begins to make the movement himself. Even if I remind him to do nothing, he continues to make precisely the same movement in response to my action. In this case, the action is too trivial to produce anxiety, and yet the pattern of tension comes into play automatically, and he moves, without even realizing he is doing so. Even more important, he seems each time to tense himself in anticipation of what I am about to do, and all because he seems preoccupied with the *idea* of what I am about to do.

This suggests a more complete answer. Richard's actions are determined not by a blind reaction, nor by his conscious intention, but by the association he has made of a movement. Consider what happens, for instance, when I tell Richard I am going to move him forward in the chair, but make a point of adding that I am *not* going to stand him up. This time, he makes the usual bracing movement in response to my moving him, pulling back his head and tightening his entire body, but instead of jumping onto his feet, he comes only as far forward in the chair as I have suggested. When, however, I say I want to move him out of the chair, and then I move him *the same distance and in the same way,* he then begins positively to jump out of the chair, even when he has agreed not to do anything.

This explains why Richard is making this unwanted action, and why it occurs against his will. If he were simply reacting because of physical tension, his actions wouldn't so accurately reflect what he knows I am about to do. But that is not the case. He unconsciously makes precisely the action I have suggested to him. This indicates that Richard is not simply doing something because of a physical tension pattern. Rather, he is unconsciously anticipating, or second-guessing, what I am about to do; and that *mental* fact explains why the tension pattern comes into play and why he performs that particular action.

The same fact explains why he lifted his arm. As I begin to raise his arm, he tries to leave it alone, but in spite of himself, he is "set" to move, and performs the action unconsciously. This action is so subtle that it is almost impossible to feel, but when I remove my hand, the arm remains in midair, demonstrating that he has in fact raised it. Again, his response is a physical pattern of tension, but it is happening because he is mentally fixated—again at a level of which he is not aware—on doing the action I have indicated I am about to do.

Richard may be convinced, then, that he has complete control over his actions, but his actions are, in a sense, at the mercy of his own thoughts. He may not want to raise his arm, but he has become preoccupied with doing that movement once I have suggested it, and he thus raises the arm in anticipation of my movement, whether he would like to or not. The most interesting aspect of the response, though, is that he does not know he has become preoccupied with raising the arm. As far as he is concerned, he is quite capable of deciding what he will or will not do; he doesn't realize that when I suggest an action, his thought process becomes dominated by the idea I have given him, at a level of which he is entirely unaware. In other words, the ideas are occurring below Richard's conscious awareness, or subconsciously.

This explains, then, why Richard's pattern of tension is so insistent, and why I am unable to stop him from harmfully tensing in response to my actions. The pattern of tension is part of an unconscious action, and that action occurs automatically once Richard gets an idea to do something. The moment I vicariously move him, at a level of which he is not aware, his knowledge of what I am about to do automatically flows into action before he even realizes it.

Richard's pattern of tension, then, isn't just tension. It is a pattern of response in which, on the one hand, a pattern of tension is set off so that an entire action will occur; and, on the other hand, in which an idea subconsciously triggers that action. Because we were initially interested in the pattern of physical tensions, we overlooked the fact that the tensions occurred as part of a larger response pattern. But once we consider the tensions from the point of view that in some cases we've asked Richard to do nothing, and yet he has unconsciously responded to what he knows I am about to do, the tensions are suddenly revealed as a response pattern that I can mentally evoke in him at a subconscious level.

We have now unearthed a much larger event underlying our original problem. In the first several chapters, we discussed how specific muscular tensions are part of a larger pattern of tension that constitutes a malcoordinated working of his body. In physical terms, the symptom is a manifestation of this overall imbalance, and in order to solve the problem, it becomes necessary to restore a generally coordinated condition by reducing these tensions and eliciting the natural organizing response of the muscular system. In Richard's case, however, these tensions couldn't be reduced, even when we vicariously performed actions for him, because they were part of a pattern of uncontrolled activity that was triggered by ideas that operate unconsciously. A larger behavioral mechanism seems to underlay all of Richard's actions, and this mechanism begins to overshadow the problem of physical tension. Once he is mentally preoccupied with an action, he subconsciously "sets" himself for activity, and this subconscious *tendency to action* is triggered by the idea of a movement to be performed. Muscle tension alone is no longer the problem, since it is triggered by ideas occurring subconsciously in the context of activity.

Once you begin to observe the pattern of tension in this way—that is, as a pattern of activity triggered by a subconscious idea—it can be detected in various everyday actions. Let's say that I tell Richard that I would like to teach him how to hold a pen without unnecessarily straining the muscles of his hand and arm, and that, in order to do this, I would like him to leave his hand relaxed while I place the pen in his hand. When I actually bring the pen toward his hand, however, he begins to stare at the pen and impulsively reaches for it, tightening his arm and shoulder, even when I have asked him not to. The same happens with speaking. When preparing to speak, Richard has a tendency to pull back his head, to gasp in breath between phrases, and to tighten his ribs—all part of his habitual pattern of tensions when he speaks. When I make some adjustments so that these habitual tensions are reduced and ask him not to take a breath before he speaks, he again reacts automatically when confronted with the actual task. Before he has even realized it, he gasps for breath in preparation to speak, unconsciously performing the action I have suggested to him.

Again, it is not just the tensions Richard can't control. The tensions are in fact part of a larger behavior that occurs subconsciously when Richard is "taken" with the idea of writing and speaking. Earlier, we observed Richard perform actions with too much tension. But now that we reduce these tensions and ask him to refrain from engaging in the actions that cause the tensions, it is clear that the tensions occur as a total response that is subconsciously motivated once he gets the idea to act.

I should point out that Richard can control his movements to some extent. He has, as we all have, normal control over his actions, certainly to the extent that he can, for instance, stop writing or deliberately relax parts of his body while writing. He can also, incidentally, simply refuse to do anything, in which case he is able to do just that. But observe what happens when I tell Richard to hold the pen very lightly and to just scribble. Initially, he is able to refrain from actually grabbing the pen; he takes it calmly and is able to write, for the moment, with little or no sign of tension in his arms, hand, and shoulder. But let him continue to write for a minute or so, and soon he is gripping the pen so tightly that his knuckles are white, he is pressing the tip of the pen onto the page, and he has tensed throughout his body as before. This indicates that, even though Richard can exercise voluntary control over his movements, this subconscious pattern is operating, just as it was when the action was triggered.

Observing this subconscious element in action, then, reveals a hidden, yet critical, cause of tension. In the beginning of this chapter we saw that when we demonstrated to Richard how to move without harmfully tensing the neck, back and legs, he perpetuated these tensions by making unnecessary and uncontrolled movements. We also saw that these actions resulted from ideas that we had suggested to him. But it is now clear that these unwanted movements are by no means accidental, that Richard has a general tendency to respond to ideas I suggest and that, far from being a coincidence, or a byproduct of tension, these actions are the inevitable result of his own tendency to react whenever he has the idea to do something.

But exactly how do these ideas operate, and why are they subconscious? We are all familiar with the notion that a passing thought or emotion can trigger a particular memory or association. We smell a familiar smell, see a familiar face, and we are reminded—sometimes without even knowing it—of an old friend, summer camp, or schooldays. This associative process is the principle on which hypnotic suggestion works. Particularly when we are relaxed, we are susceptible to associations, which can in turn evoke physical action. We don't know all the thoughts, or connections between thoughts, that exist in the brain, but they constantly influence our waking life without our being conscious, because that is their function.

We are susceptible to movement in a similar way. If, for instance, we hear a particular sound, it doesn't consciously occur to us that the sound is significant. It is only when we are responding to the sound that we realize a fire alarm has gone off. In other words, the subconscious link between one thought and another is capable of triggering a particular action.

When I suggested the act of standing to Richard, the same mental process was in operation, and it allowed me to evoke particular responses in him. Although, at a particular moment, he may resist what I ask of him, or choose to do something else, it is nevertheless inevitable that, in simply listening to what I say, he is going to be influenced by what I suggest, even if he chooses not to be. If Richard knows from my words or movements that I intend to move him into a standing position, or to lift his arm, he will be susceptible to that action, because he has mentally associated what I am doing with standing or raising the arm, at a level of which he is not aware.

When you understand the various elements in this phenomenon, you can literally evoke an action in someone, simply by knowing how to get him or her mentally fixated on that activity. Lifting Richard's arm is a case in point. If you do not tell him what you are about to do, and very quickly raise his arm, he may not raise it, because he has no thought of doing so. But if you explain to him that in fact you intend to raise his arm and would prefer that he not assist in any way by raising the arm himself, then his very intention not to make the action will fixate him on the movement, and the moment he realizes you are trying to raise his arm—and sometimes even before you have raised it—he will impulsively perform the action, subconsciously responding to the idea you have suggested to him. When this happens, he will probably not be aware it has happened, but if you let go of his arm, he will readily see that he has in fact raised it, because it will remain in midair by itself.

You have thus demonstrated the suggestion, or mental factor, in action.

In spite of his intention not to move his arm, Richard raises (and holds) it because your asking him not to do so has evoked the idea of raising it, which brought about the action, unconsciously performed. Usually the "subject" is unaware of this phenomenon and how it operates. If, for instance, you point out to Richard that he had intended not to make this action, he may object by saying that, on the contrary, he had intended to do so. By simply asking him to do nothing, however, you can easily test his claim. If he agrees to your request, and raises the arm the next time you move it in spite of his agreement, then you have positive proof that the action was an automatic—or subconscious—response to your suggestion. I should point out that this action is not easy to reproduce if you do not know how to move someone in a way that associates with a particular action—that is, if you do not know how to evoke the desired association. It is also possible for the "subject" to resist what you are doing by simply doing something entirely different, although this will work only if the determination to do nothing is stronger than the idea of moving. Nevertheless, the propensity to act is so great that even when the subject resists, the action is often evoked against his will. The interesting feature in this entire process is that although you ask him not to do anything, the suggestion has precisely the opposite effect, since the request not to do something suggests not the idea of nothing but the very movement the subject is trying not to perform! In fact, if you ask the subject to deliberately refrain from performing a movement, that movement is often even more likely to occur, since the subject's efforts not to perform the movement will reinforce his subconscious fixation on the act itself, thus making it even more difficult *not* to think about the action.

However, the action is not a *direct* response to the association. If it were, Richard would jump out of the chair the moment he knew I wanted to stand him up or, for that matter, whenever he thought of *any* action. This would mean he would be making irrelevant movements all the time—a dangerous tendency that is countered, in evolutionary development, by the ability to withhold from action, to choose wisely from among crucial alternatives. In fact, the suggestion determines the course of the action once the action takes place, but some further stimulus is required for the idea to actually discharge into activity—in this case, my moving him. In this sense, there are two elements operating: first, the mental association, which is registered subconsciously, and second, the response itself, which takes place only when I actually begin to move Richard.

It is also interesting to note that when Richard has become familiar with this tendency, he will soon be able, to some extent, to resist it. If when I raise his arm he is able to make his arm go "heavy," he will find that instead of reacting to what I have done, he will have managed to prevent the raising of the arm. But the original tendency is by no means eradicated. Later in the learning process, when the tendency to collapse or relax is reduced by improving his physical coordination, it will be clear that, instead of doing nothing, Richard is now positively collapsing downward in response to my suggestion. It is possible, in other words, to supplant one tendency with another; but the new tendency is simply another version of a subconscious action, this time more disguised than before.

It is also important to note that although it is possible to "plant" an idea in someone's head and thus artificially trigger actions in that person, the desire to initiate action on our own provides the natural, or usual, source of these associations. If instead of vicariously moving Richard, I ask him to stand up on his own, this time it will appear that he is performing the action simply because he wants to. But closer observation reveals otherwise. If I ask Richard to again stand on his own, but to initiate the movement slowly, it is not difficult to observe how impulsively he stands on his feet the moment he thinks of standing. He is again being "triggered" into action, but this time the action is a response to his own idea of standing, which triggers the muscles into activity and causes the action to happen, just as when I moved him.

Although it is thus possible to trigger Richard artificially into action, the tendency is ever-present, and the reason is that this mechanism explains the normal process by which Richard gets the idea to do something, and then does it. We have only to see that small gasp of breath when beginning to speak, that small impulsive movement at the moment of standing up, and we know that Richard's own actions are in fact motivated by the same subconscious process that governs the actions we involuntarily triggered in him a moment earlier. When we trigger Richard into activity, this event is in fact an artificial case of a normal pro cess; voluntary action happens in precisely the same way and for the same reasons: as a reaction to his own mental association, or idea, of an action to be performed.

The normal occurrence of ideas that lead to actions also explains why the triggered actions aren't simply a blind reaction, or an involuntary response, to being moved. If action is a response to a mental association, and if mental associations normally trigger voluntary actions, then we know that what appears to be an involuntary response is in fact based on the same pattern of activity as voluntary action and so isn't involuntary at all. What appears to be a reaction, in other words, is motivated by a complex and subtle mechanism—usually called voluntary behavior—in which ideas trigger actions.

I said earlier that I wanted to introduce the mental dimension involved in the pattern of physical tension, and we can now begin to amend our original conception of the problem to include this mental element. In the first several chapters we observed a physical pattern of tension, and knowing how the system naturally can lengthen, we saw how it could be rectified to allow for a more complete and integrated activity. Seeing the problem this way, we concluded that there was a physical problem, and we identified it as a harmful pattern of tension that interfered, in movement and at rest, with the normal operation of this basic mechanism. From this point of view, it was perfectly natural that we should view the problem as a physical one, because that was our interest and focus.

We now see, though, that this point of view wasn't entirely accurate. The physical pattern occurs as action in response to mental associations, and this is the true context within which it operates. In this sense, the pattern of tension is really an abstraction from a larger whole of which it is a part—a complex mental and physical process that must be clearly understood if this pattern is to be brought under conscious control.

Ideo-Motor Action

In the last section, we set out to identify the mental component in physical actions. Our initial difficulty led us to discover a tension pattern that interfered with our innate physical muscular mechanism. This explained, at the physical level, the cause of muscular tension and strain. The next step was to understand what caused the tension pattern. By attempting to prevent this tension in activity, we saw that it was elicited at a subconscious level by the idea of performing actions.

The moment we uncover the larger behavioral pattern in which muscular activity is triggered subconsciously, however, we have a number of new problems to explain. It is well known that there are subtle connections between mind and body; in this sense, we can understand that muscles, movements, and gestures would be susceptible to ideas and attitudes. This does not, however, explain the function of such a connection, or make sense of its structure. Why should it be the case that muscular activity is susceptible to associative processes? Why do these ideas operate, and why are they communicated subconsciously? What is the relationship between the unwanted actions we have observed, and conscious, voluntary activity?

This will be the subject of this and the following chapters. It is common, in the mind/body field, to speak of practices that give relief for various ailments. Usually these practices describe methods for relaxing the mind, enhancing immune function, and the like. But because these methods are focused on producing immediate effects, they do not place the symptoms in a larger context and so fail to articulate exactly what the problem is. The problem of muscular tension, however, falls squarely within the field of psychology—the psychology of how action takes place; and this is a crucial aspect of the problem that must be understood and described before we try to outline solutions or practices for dealing with the problem.

We saw a moment ago that when Richard performed an action, the pattern of tension was in fact linked to ideas and could be triggered by them. At first it appeared that when Richard moved, he could decide how the movement could take place and could therefore prevent the harmful tensions that accompanied the movement. But he was not, in fact, able to deliberately control his own actions, because these actions were the result of mental associations that triggered the actions at a subconscious level.

This role of associations in action represents a critical element in

Richard's problem. Up to this point, we have found that muscular tension is triggered by ideas that occur at a subconscious level. Because tension is physical in nature, the physical side of the problem was naturally the aspect which concerned us, and so we took an interest in the mental dimension of the problem only insofar as it related to the triggering of the physical tension. What was not clear, however, was why the muscles and ideas were linked, until we observed their underlying role in virtually all of Richard's actions. Normally, we think the mind is in some way in command of the body; in this sense we make a separation between mind and body. But the real nature of ideas and muscles is that they are linked in our voluntary behavior, and this explains the true nature of actions and how they take place.

Consider, for instance, what happens when you take a pen in your hand and begin writing. The decision to write is made, but it is not separate from the response of the body. The idea and the act form a seamless whole. This is in fact how all voluntary action takes place. An idea—in Richard's case, the idea to speak, to lift his arm, or to stand—produces a motor effect, the two elements occurring as one event. These ideas, as we saw, operate mostly subconsciously—that is, automatically and unthinkingly. But the main point is that action issues from thought, the two being, for all intents and purposes, continuous. Both elements are part of a physical and mental mechanism that is designed to work this way. When we asked Richard to speak without gasping, he hesitated at first, trying not to take a breath in preparation to speak. But when he subconsciously thought of speaking, he gasped in preparation to speak in spite of his intention, because the idea of speaking triggered the motor activity.

This explains why ideas connect with muscular activity, and what the function of this connection is. When we perform an action, we have the subjective sense that we have somehow "told" our body what to do, that our mind, or ego, is in charge of the body. In this sense, we make a distinct separation between the mind and the body. In fact, there is no such separation, and the feeling that there is one belies the reality of how we actually perform voluntary actions. You are sitting, reading a book, and then decide to go to the kitchen to get something to drink. However, the "decision" to get up is not so much a conscious process as an associative flow of ideas into action. We feel afterwards that we "did" the action; we have a sense that we commanded the act, that we controlled it. But the action was largely a mechanical process in which mental events led to a physical, or motor, act at a subconscious level of which we are almost entirely unaware.

The reason, then, why Richard has ideas, why he is suggestible, and why these ideas operate so fluidly is because this process is the means by which all voluntary action happens. When I run to catch the bus, I may subjectively feel that my mind, my ego, is commanding my body to run. A bit of introspection, however, reveals that the moment I saw the bus, this idea set into motion a train of associations—most of which I am not even aware of—and I find that I am running before I have even "decided" to act. I don't get up to answer the phone because of a conscious choice so much as because I associate the ring with the need to find out who is calling. And I don't write at my desk because I have decided to pick up a pen so much as because I have remembered that I need to write a letter, and I find myself walking into my office to find pen and paper. Most of our actions are, like my reaction to seeing the bus or my needing to write a letter, fluid, unthinking responses to thoughts that trigger these actions.

This concept of how ideas flow into motor acts is not new to psychology. William James, in *The Principles of Psychology* (1890), debunks the notion of a mysterious *will* that oversees actions; in most cases, James asserts, action simply flows out of associations of thought. This conception in James's work was a challenge to the commonly held belief that our actions issue from our conscious will—that we choose to do things, and that what we have done we have chosen to do. The vast majority of our actions, James argues, are not "chosen" at all, in the sense that we usually mean, but issue "upon the mere thought of it" (James 1890b:522). Action, or motor activity, is linked with thought, and since our thoughts follow associational paths, the action which flows from thought is dictated strictly by causal laws. James, borrowing the term from earlier writers, called this phenomenon *ideo-motor action*.

* The term "ideo-motor" action actually originated with William Carpenter, a 19th century physiologist. In his *Principles of Mental Physiology* (1887) he challenges the view that actions follow the dictates of the will, and on the basis of this concept explains everyday behaviors as well as unexplained phenomena that, he says, are in fact automatic forms of action.

To take an example, I am washing a dish in the kitchen, and once it is clean I find that I am rinsing the dish under the water and then reaching a moment later for the saucepan. I do not know exactly how each movement occurred. But the situational context sets off associations that issue in motor acts, which then trigger other associations and actions, all of which are habitually learned and mostly automatic. (See Figure 5.)

If such a view were not true, how could we account for the remarkable fact that we can perform all the actions of everyday life so automatically? Washing our hands, walking to the store, cooking a meal—

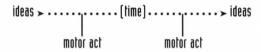

Figure 5
Ideas and motor acts

these are incredibly complex activities, and we couldn't possibly think about each and every one. We do them, in fact, unthinkingly and without any consciousness of their difficulty. It is precisely this ideo-motor function that accounts for them. James writes:

> ...*all the ingrained procedures by which life is carried on—the manners and customs, dressing and undressing, acts of salutation, etc.—are executed in this semi-automatic way unhesitatingly and efficiently, the very outermost margin of consciousness seeming to be concerned in them, while the focus may be occupied with widely different things (James 1950:117-18).*

However, James points out, there are many cases in which we deliberately choose to do one thing as opposed to another, or where no action results from our thought at all. James illustrates his point by describing the dilemma that is created by conflicting desires—that of waking up in the morning and deciding whether to turn over and go back to sleep or to get up. In this case, "the motor consequences of the first idea (getting out of bed) are blocked," producing a deadlock. This situation is resolved in one of two ways:

> *(1) I may forget for a moment the thermometric conditions, and the idea of getting up will immediately discharge into act; I shall suddenly find that I have got up—or*

> *(2) still mindful of the freezing temperature, the thought of the duty of rising may become so pungent that it determines action in spite of inhibition. In the latter case, I have a sense of energetic moral effort, and consider that I have done a virtuous act (James: 1950:119).*

The choice, however, does not issue from "an express fiat of will," but represents a resolution of the existing pathways that are already, in a sense, in competition. These competing possibilities represent a more complex field of consciousness than exists in the case of simple unimpeded associations. Choice, as James explains above, consists in the relaxing of one idea or the intensification of the other, so that a particular idea wins out in the conflict between the competing aims within the field of ideas. "All cases of willful action properly so called," James writes, "of choice after hesitation and deliberation, may be conceived after one of these latter patterns" (James 1950:119).

Even when we do one particular thing, then, as opposed to another, our will is not a "superior agent" that imposes itself upon our behavior independently of existing associative pathways. All behavior—even when our conscious will has intervened—is a complicated version of motor action issuing from ideas. It is the fact that one idea wins out in a complicated field of ideas that creates the illusion of choice. This complex field of ideas also explains why we are not continually responding to ideas. The continual competition of ideas cancels or inhibits the discharge of most of these ideas into activity, which is why the flow of mental associations does not appear to have a direct link to action. "The reason why [the doctrine of ideo-motor action] is not a self-evident truth," James writes, "is because we have so many ideas which *do not* result in action" (James 1890b:525).

Action, then, operates according to the mental law of association, and this process explains why these associations are mostly subconscious. When we think about something, we usually conceive this process in terms of conscious will, or consciousness. But in fact most of our associations are not conscious, but occur below our level of awareness. When I "decide" to walk to the kitchen, I don't normally review the various reasons for doing so; they occur naturally as a process of interconnecting associations that are part of my ongoing memory of what is in the kitchen, my need to eat, and so on. The vast majority of our actions result from just such a subconscious process of association. Most action is in fact an unthinking, automatic response to what is happening around us, within the context of the many stimuli that make up our everyday environment.

This associative process also explains how voluntary action can take place even within the confines of such a deterministic process. Although the process by which associations take place is a deterministic one, it is the fact of having associations, not the fact that I am conscious, that makes for choice. The phone rings, and I find myself walking toward it. But if while I am walking to the phone, I spot a dollar bill on the floor, I will alter my course of action and kneel down to retrieve it instead of continuing to the kitchen. Actions follow a predictable routine of associations, but the possibilities of associations are what account for choice. Choice, in most cases, results not from my ability to consciously think about what I want to do but from the flexible exercise of choice among the various possibilities created by the associations I can have.

This explains, then, how our actions, which so much feel to us as if they emanate from our will, can at the same time be "determined" responses. Our acts are not just initiated out of thin air by "consciousness," but are themselves a subtle kind of response, a delicate interplay of thought and motor activity. Action occurs as thought, and to say there is action is to say that there is thinking going on. Our usual assumption is that our behavior is willed—a pointer that we can aim at our desired ends in order to carry out our chosen actions. But what appears to be willed is in fact the result of ideas, a subtle response to our own mental associations.

The key, then, to the subconscious pattern of triggering we observed in Richard in the last section is the ideo-motor pattern of activity, and this provides a critical piece in understanding the larger context within which the harmful pattern of tension operates. I said in the beginning that when we observe physical tension, we characterize it as physical because it is so directly related to the body and movement. When we saw, in the last chapter, how much this phenomenon was in fact mental in nature, this nevertheless did not explain why it was there. We can now understand the pattern of tension in its true context. The tension pattern is in fact part of a larger whole in which ideas and muscles function together in the context of action, and this explains why the tension occurs as part of the total ideo-motor pathway.

It is important to note, though, that the "motor act" to which James refers is not, strictly speaking, the same as the tension pattern we have observed. The act of getting out of bed in the morning (or getting out of a chair or speaking) is an overt act; this is what James refers to as a motor act. The pattern of tension, in contrast, is the machinery that brings about this overt act. Reducing this tension makes it possible to gain increased control over the motor act.

Bringing about a condition of reduced tension, then, alters the organic conditions which influence the ideo-motor action mechanism, and this is essential to gaining control over the overt act. In his account of ideo-motor action, James was not trying to solve the practical problem of how to improve physical functioning but simply combatting the assumption that a mysterious "will" is responsible for action. As a result, he did not describe, in any detail, the machinery of ideo-motor action, or whether there is anything wrong with this machinery. Accordingly, he gives no account of the bodily mechanics underlying the phenomenon. For him, to use an analogy, the mechanism of ideo-motor action is like that of a car. By pressing the gas pedal, ideo-motor action can be put into motion (the idea) and it can be driven a certain distance (overt motor act), but what goes on under the hood—the machinery itself—is omitted. He takes it for granted that the engine is there to work, to carry out the particular actions necessary, because, like a well-running engine, the body is designed to produce movement and doesn't need attention.

In examining the machinery of ideo-motor action, however, we have taken a direct interest, not only in the idea and motor act, but in the way in which the machinery itself is working—we have looked under the hood, as it were, to see how the car is running. Ideas may somehow produce motor outcomes, but there is a mechanism—the muscular system—that accounts for the motor outcome. At the moment Richard gets an idea, we can feel an increase in tension, a pulling back of the head, a tightening of the neck, an arching of the back—all happening in direct response to a subconscious mental association. In short, we see the way in which the engine works, the actual moving of parts that results in the completed motor act. In this sense, the problem of tension isn't simply physical but represents the organic aspect of the total pathway of activity that is itself working incorrectly. This led us to locate the engine under the hood, the actual machinery that goes into gear for the accomplishing of acts such as getting out of bed, picking up a pen, or speaking.

When this tension pattern is reduced, however, and when the use of the muscular system is improved in activity, then this organic condition is dramatically altered. Because the tensions represent not simply how an action is performed but the organic basis of the ideo-motor mechanism itself, then the possibility of awareness and control of the ideo-motor response is thereby increased. How the act is performed alters the possibility of what happens in the act itself. In this sense, physical changes must precede mental ones, because the organic conditions on which the ideo-motor pathway depends are basic to the pathway of behavior. The mind, so often conceived as a function that controls the body, cannot be quickened without first altering organic, or bodily, conditions; and awareness, which is usually regarded as the basis for change, must follow, not precede, the change in organic conditions.

Understanding the tension pattern as the machinery of the ideo-motor response, however, is still only part of the problem. When we triggered Richard into an action, we saw that he subconsciously reacts to what I am doing by performing that action himself. We thought at first that this response was purely physical, until we later saw it as a total response, and linked it with ideo-motor action. But what would happen if we could get him to prevent this tension from occurring—that is, to make the same action, but without tensing the neck muscles, arching the back, and so on? At first glance, it would appear that the only difference would be the lessened amount of tension and the correspondingly increased efficiency of the movement. But the tension *is* the response; when Richard is able to notice and prevent the pulling back of the head, he doesn't actually jump out of the chair as before, but is able to prevent the response entirely. In other words, the tension is itself connected with the response— so much so that when the tension is prevented he is no longer susceptible to being triggered into action.

This reveals another crucial aspect of the problem. All voluntary action involves a connection of thought to muscular action, running along a nervous circuit which we might describe as mental and neurological as well as physical, since ideas and muscles connect *via* a nervous pathway. This fact holds true even when Richard does not indulge in the unnecessary tension, since coordinated movement, as we saw earlier, does not involve the unnecessary or harmful pattern of tension. When Richard tenses in preparation for movement, though, something more is happening. As I move him over his feet, he jumps out of the chair, even when he doesn't want to; he grabs the pen even when he is trying to relax his arm. The pattern of tension, then, isn't necessary to this normal nervous activity, but implies a change in the propensity for that action to occur, and in the intensity of the action when it does occur. In other words, the presence of the tension pattern indicates that the pathway of activity is more excitable and that the ideo-motor circuit is therefore more susceptible to being triggered than if the tension weren't present.

To say that the tension pattern represents the machinery of the ideo-motor response, then, isn't entirely accurate. Muscular action is necessary to the overt motor act; in this sense, muscular action is the machinery of ideo-motor action. But since the triggered action doesn't occur without the tension, the tension pattern represents the machinery not of the ideo-motor response but of its "wrong" working. And this wrong working is characterized, not simply by the increased level of tension, but by the susceptibility to activity that accompanies it.

Ideo-motor action, then, does not require the presence of harmful tensions to operate normally, and this is as it should be. How can a normal function (ideo-motor action) be explained by an abnormal function (the harmful pattern of tension)? We began by observing the tension pattern because it was harmful, and this led us, in turn, to uncover its connection with ideas in activity. But we should certainly not be satisfied with the concept of ideo-motor action if it can only be explained on the basis of harmful tensions that are not in fact present in animals and young children, in whom the ideo-motor function is fully intact. The only way out of this difficulty is to consider whether the harmful tension is, in fact, an extraneous element in the equation. In fact, that is precisely the case. The pattern of tension, as we've seen, represents a variation on the theme of normal ideo-motor action, and that is precisely what makes ideo-motor action, in the present context, so significant. Without such a concept, we simply cannot fully explain the problem of tension. It is interesting to consider, however, that although ideo-motor action normally operates without the presence of a harmful pattern of tension, it would not have been possible to discover its role in the present context unless the tension pattern had been present. The abnormality of the ideo-motor responses in Richard highlights the less noticeable subtleties of normal ideo-motor action. From the point of view of our present study, then, the wrong working of the ideo-motor response has made it possible to identify what is normal by virtue of accentuating elements that would otherwise have been disguised.

This last fact is the key to our discussion and uncovers yet another layer of the problem. I said in the beginning that the study of the problem of tension and stress involves a complicated mental and physical whole; we began to observe this psychophysical whole by linking the observable pattern of tension to a circuit, or pathway, of association and motor act that is clearly mental and physical. But identifying such a connection does not prove that the disturbance in this mechanism is both physical and mental. It is well known in physiology that all acts are psychophysical, but this does not mean that all forms of physical pathology indicate the presence of mental pathology as well. To say that physical acts are part of a psychophysical whole does not help us to understand the tension pattern any more than if we had remained with our original assumption that the problem was purely physical.

But we are not simply noting a physical problem and then observing that it is connected with the mind. We saw that there is a tension pattern and that it is connected with associations in action. But this linkage, which represents normal motor function, is triggered unnecessarily. This means that not only the physical machinery but the unified mental and physical working of this mechanism, is in some sense disturbed. The tension pattern we have observed is the physical aspect of nothing less than a wrong working of the ideo-motor mechanism, whereby the response to the idea to do something is too readily triggered by thought.

We can now identify what is wrong, both physically and mentally, within the context of this working mechanism, or at least begin to do so. Muscular action is not separate from activity but part of it. The muscular system is in some sense responsive to thought; this is how action takes place. This means that the pattern of tension isn't simply a feature of movement but part of the mechanism of activity itself. When Richard pulls back his head and braces in preparation to move, this muscular activity is triggered by the thought of moving; but the tightening and bracing represent a tendency to be more susceptible to be triggered into activity than should normally be the case. The tension, then, can be said to be part of a total pattern of response that has two sides. On the one hand, there is the physical, or motor, aspect. This is observable as the actual response, the completed motor act; it is also the aspect that we "see" most clearly. Less obvious is the mental aspect, or the way we receive a stimulus. We usually think of this aspect in terms of a will or ego that commands the body to act; but as we have seen, action includes a receptive component: the ability to respond to influences from within the mind and from outside in the form of mental associations that are elicited by experience. (See Figure 6.)

These two aspects constitute ideo-motor action as a mental and physical process; the pattern of tension is part of this total process. And because both aspects of this pathway are imbalanced, it is not just the physical action that is harmful, but the working of ideo-motor action as a total behavioral mechanism. As I will show later in more detail, this involves a complication and disturbance in the mental and physical elements involved in this function, as well as a harmful and uncontrolled ten-

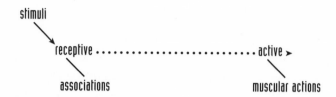

Figure 6
Receptive and active spectrum of stimulus-response pattern

dency in behavior. The pattern of tension we have observed in Richard's action, then, is not simply associated with a larger physiological process that involves mental and nervous activity but represents a disturbance in this physiological process itself. As we have seen, it is easy to assume that this problem is purely physical, for the reasons that made the mental aspect so hard to perceive to begin with. Tension is tension, pure and simple. Other factors (such as emotional stress) seem to impinge upon this physical condition, not because tension is itself part of a unified mental and physical function, but because emotions seem to "manifest" in the body. But when we perceive tension as an aspect of a total pathway and can clearly identify how this pathway operates, then it becomes clear that the physical pattern occurs within the context of a larger behavioral function that includes a mental component that operates subconsciously, the two being for all intents and purposes an inseparable whole. It is this fact that explains why we could produce an action in Richard by suggesting it, and why the tension is therefore part of a larger pattern of activity.

We can now see the total problem in a nutshell. We first observed a pattern of tension, which we later discovered to be part of a larger mechanism, a total circuitry in which mental and physical factors operate to produce action. Knowing now that the tension was part of this ideo-motor response, we could see that the machinery is itself working incorrectly. By then testing the pattern of action, we could observe that, when the tension pattern was eliminated, it was more difficult to elicit the response. This indicated that although the triggered action was an example of ideo-motor action, the tension that made it possible to trigger Richard out of the chair represented something wrong in the working, not just of the physical mechanism, but of this total circuitry—a propensity for it to go into activity too easily.

The problem of tension, and its interference with the reflexive working of the postural system (to return to our original problem), can now be seen very clearly as a problem that falls clearly within the realm of psychology. At the beginning of this section, we observed that, although we could see a link between subconscious ideas and physical tension, we still didn't know the reason for this connection. We can now say with some certainty what this psychological process is. Ideas link with motor acts in the process of producing behavior; the problem of tension sits squarely in the context of this ideo-motor function.

Action and Reaction

A few moments ago I said that when we perform an action we subjectively feel that we have "willed" ourselves to move, when in fact the action is the result of mental associations which flow unconsciously into activity. We found this by observing in a way we would not normally do: by looking first at a pattern of physical movement and then noting its connection with mental activity in producing that action. This led us to understand how as a mechanism the mental and physical aspects work together in the form of ideo-motor action, and how that mechanism of activity is in fact working incorrectly.

This began to provide a critical piece in understanding the origins of problems that, in the mind/body field, we perceive as physical. Initially, we observed a harmful tension pattern, and we saw how this tension interfered with the muscular system. Removing the tension allowed this system to work normally. But this apparently physical problem was, in fact, intimately connected with activity. Once we established that relationship, the problem shifted from correcting an imbalance in the muscular system to preventing subconscious activity that perpetuates that interference.

This shift in perspective begins to alter how we look at the mind and body. We saw that when Richard tensed himself during simple movements, this tension was part of a larger pattern of activity that could be subconsciously triggered into action when he was given the idea of doing something. But we also saw that these triggered actions were artificial instances of how action normally takes place. When Richard walks across the room, answers the phone, or writes a letter, these actions, although voluntary, are equally the result of his own, mostly subconscious, associations. To some degree, then, Richard's normal voluntary actions are just another form of the earlier case in which we triggered him automatically into activity. In these cases, he would say (and he would be right) that he had the intention to perform these actions. But even these voluntary actions, because they occur automatically in response to associations, are in some sense reactive and unconscious.

This similarity between triggered movements and ones that Richard makes deliberately begins to blur the distinction between what is voluntary and what is involuntary, and this in turn begins to reveal assumptions we make about the mind and body. Even when we accept in theory the idea that action is the result of a complex mental and physical process that is largely unconscious, we still reserve a special place for our own voluntary conduct, which we feel is somehow commanded by a controlling mind. When we observe someone going to work, cooking a meal, or speaking on the phone, we don't, after all, "see" a mental and physical mechanism operating, but a person: we have a sense of an ego, a personality, that is in command. The fact is, whatever we might think about psychophysical unity or about the neurophysiology of human behavior, we hold fast to the assumption that behavior—whether ours or that of another—is largely the result of an inner personality.

But most physical actions simply aren't the result of an autonomous ego. Consider, as another example, what happens when Richard engages in a conversation with a group of people. He has a subjective sense that he speaks because he chooses to, but time after time we can observe him unable to wait until the other person has finished speaking and, noticeably gasping in breath when he hears something he disagrees with or wants to challenge, erupt into speech. In this case, of course, we could say that his action was a reaction, but where exactly does one draw the line between voluntary action and involuntary reaction? Virtually every voluntary action Richard makes is, like his act of reacting to someone else during a conversation, as much a reaction to something as it is a voluntary action emanating from his own inner will, and knowing this makes it increasingly difficult to identify the "agent" of personality, or mind, that governs these actions. (See Figure 7.)

The notion, then, that an autonomous ego governs our actions is an illusion, and it belies the true nature of our physical actions. Imagine a crab, which you are observing through an underwater camera, moving about on the floor of the ocean. Its behavior appears fluid, intelligent, and well adapted to its surroundings as it hides from prey or searches for food. If, however, you remove the crab from its surroundings and hold it in midair while it continues to frantically and mechanically move its legs, the same actions that appeared so purposive, or cognitively rational, now appear rather robotic and ludicrous.

We make similar assumptions about human behavior. Whatever we may learn from physiology or psychology, we subjectively feel ourselves to be autonomous and, therefore, when we observe others, we impute this same power to them. The body may be capable of knee-jerk responses,

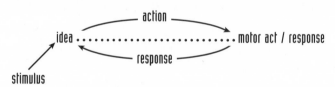

Figure 7
The continuum of action and reaction

but we put behavior—that is, our daily actions or conduct—in a different category entirely, and this category remains for the most part immune to much of what science has to say. But once we begin to examine Richard's actions close-up, once we begin to experiment with his behavior by separating his actions from their normal context, then, as with the crab, we can perceive how action occurs with a more objective eye.

That, in a nutshell, is what we have done in the previous sections. By "removing" Richard from his usual surroundings, we are able to discern uncontrolled elements in his behavior that would otherwise appear to be deliberate and rational. Actions that appear to emanate from an autonomous personality are in fact as much a reaction, an automatic pattern of muscular activity that happens in response to his own mental associations, as they are self-directed. And since these responses occur even when Richard is trying *not* to do anything, think how much more powerfully they must operate when he is actively engaged in daily activities. The routine acts of everyday life—getting on a bus, answering the phone, bending to pick something up—happen so quickly and unthinkingly that their automatic nature is even more difficult to perceive than in the artificial cases we have looked at. But if, as in Richard's case, we could slow each action down and observe its origin, we would be struck to observe how many actions are in fact triggered subconsciously, and how these actions occur as a pattern of muscular action that is triggered continually by the various stimuli presented by daily life.

Once we look at human behavior in this way, it becomes virtually impossible to divorce the study of tension and movement from voluntary action and "mind." It is common today to speak of the "mind/body connection"; more recently, researchers have shown how the mind "talks" to the body through the media of peptides and other chemicals that are transmitted by the brain whenever we have a passing thought or an emotion. But when we observe the intimate connection between muscular tension and actions that are set in motion by ideas, it becomes apparent that because this way of speaking is preserving the distinction of mind and body, current mind/body concepts cannot do justice to the practical reality of becoming aware of the causes of tension and stress. The very idea of a mind that speaks to the body, or that influences physical functioning, is itself a dualistic concept that doesn't adequately reflect the way in which bodily movement and ideas operate as a unified whole in action, and therefore is inadequate to address the problem of everyday stress and tension to which these concepts are often applied.

This assumption of a mind/body split is often attributed to the dualism of Descartes and to the ancient Greek philosophers, who began to conceptualize the material world, or the body, as fundamentally distinct from the immaterial world, which they related to abstract concepts and the ability to think. But even more basic than culturally inherited attitudes, more basic than anything we learn or are shown, are the assumptions arising from personal, subjective experience. From an early age, we experience ourselves as agents capable of willful action; we subjectively experience ourselves as an ego that commands the body. This subjective perception creates a constellation of the most ingrained preconceptions: that action is created by a mind that has power over the body; that the body is somehow separate from the mind; and that there is, inside each person, a kind of inner personality that governs action and that accounts for each and every action that takes place.

This preconception has a flip side. If there is a mind that oversees action, then the body that obeys—and that sometimes doesn't because the body is so fallible—occupies another domain—the domain of body, instinct, and reaction. When, for instance, we observed the pattern of tension, we designated this phenomenon as predominantly physical, so much so that we tended to overlook the essential role that thinking played in the movement. Behavior is seen as emanating from a personality; tension is therefore placed in the domain of the body. If we go so far as to say that tension is related to the mind, the relation is again conceived in terms of two separate parts that communicate, or interact.

The same is true when we move Richard and he involuntarily jumps out of the chair. In this case, his action is clearly behavioral in some general sense. Yet to most observers, this response has little to do with voluntary behavior as such, but appears, instead, to be a startle response, an uncontrolled reaction—a not entirely unwarranted assumption in the case of jumping so uncontrollably onto one's feet. Nevertheless, this assumption arises from the same preconception: when we work at a desk, drive to work, or make a phone call, we have the subjective conviction that these actions are overseen by the personality, the ego, and are therefore entirely voluntary. Automatic reactions, in contrast, therefore belong to the domain of the body, of instinctive reaction and impulse. When we test such assumptions through experimentation, however, it becomes clear that this is a false distinction, and that it arises in large part out of the bias that the body and physical action are separate from the mind or ego. What appears to be a reaction is in fact how Richard speaks and acts all the time—on the phone, at work, walking down the street—except that in an artificial context the action is sufficiently impulsive that we do not associate it with voluntary behavior. In short, the action that appears to be a physical reaction involves the same process, the same thoughts and muscular activity, as voluntary actions that take place in the context of everyday behavior.

The notions, then, of a mind that oversees the body and of a body that obeys it are in fact wrong, and they express a dualistic attitude that amounts to a kind of cultural prejudice. When we observe someone's behavior, we assume that the behavior emanates from the will, and that this will, having power over the body, is separate from it. When we observe movement, or the concrete muscular act of doing something, we assume we're looking at muscles, at physical action, not at the expression of someone's personality in the form of voluntary action. But both notions—that of the autonomous ego separate from the body, and that of the body separate from the mind—are mystifications or abstractions. It is perfectly acceptable to speak of the body as a system, as when we speak of circulation or digestion, or describe the postural muscles and how they support the body against gravity. It is also acceptable, when referring to cognitive activity or personality attributes, to speak of a "mind" that is in some sense separate from the body. But where the practical problem of muscle tension and stress are concerned, there is no such thing as a "body," nor is activity the result of some kind of inner "mind." To speak of both is mind/body dualism in the worst sense of the word, and it creates a rift that once made is impossible to bridge and which in practice means barren theory and ineffective practice. In the present context, mind and body constitute one whole, and they operate together in the form of a unified pathway of activity. To conceive muscle activity in terms of its connection with mental activity, and voluntary action in terms of its connection with muscular activity, is to conceive of a true psychology of action—a psychology based on a unified concept of mind and body.

Understanding the false dichotomy of mind and body makes it possible to arrive at a truly practical understanding of mind and body. Biology, physiology, medical science, and other modern scientific disciplines have given us a worldview of the human being as a biological entity whose mental and physical processes are inseparable. But this perception rarely extends, in any practical way, into the practical domain of our understanding of the mind and body as a living, functioning organism. Recognizing that tension and stress relate to lifestyle, mental attitude, and emotions, we are content with stress-reduction techniques that appeal to the link between mind and body as the basis for providing a theory of stress. But "mind" and "body" relate to the process of activity itself, and it is not possible to address fully the connection between the two by practicing methods that produce therapeutic results but which do not provide an educational means of gaining an awareness and control of this activity in living. Even when scientific research is brought to bear on the problem of stress, the methods that are based on such empirical evidence rarely deal with the problem of behavior itself. By creating the illusion that the problem can be addressed by means of therapeutic techniques, they end up reinforcing the separation between mind and body. The rift between mind and body is then repeated in the form of a division between the subjective world of everyday volition and behavior, and the world of objective scientific investigation. Such "objective" observations and methods for reducing tension and stress simply cannot provide a real understanding of the human being as a living process, or provide a truly educational approach to the problem of the control of behavior.

The problem that must ultimately be solved if we are to remove the symptoms associated with Richard's behavior is the control of behavior itself. Real mind/body unity implies a living process whereby the mental and physical aspects of action are related, not as distinct entities that indirectly influence or communicate to each other, but as descriptive aspects of the same event. Because this activity occurs subconsciously, the challenge that this event poses is the fundamental educational problem of how to raise this process to a conscious level.

Ideo-Motor Action in Relation to Physical Problems

We have now looked in some detail at how the pattern of muscular tension is linked with mental ideas to produce action. Let us look now at the relation of ideo-motor action to physical problems, beginning with the practical problem of how to prevent the ideo-motor pattern. We saw earlier that in all his actions Richard's muscular system was tensing incor-

rectly, and that this pattern of tension interfered with the normal working of his muscular system as a whole. In order to address this problem,
it was necessary to make various adjustments, restoring a more coordinated overall condition. As we saw, however, it was not sufficient simply to restore the body to its lengthened condition, since the tension
pattern recurred in activity. The key, as we saw, was to maintain this
reduced tension while assisting Richard in performing habitual actions
in a new way.

As we saw, however, preventing the ideo-motor response was not an
easy matter. We saw first that if I asked Richard to move without tensing his back, his idea to do the act—even if he intended not to tighten
or shorten while moving—invoked the ideo-motor pattern, and he would
perform the act as he always had—by tensing the back and indulging in
the usual pattern. In order to prevent this response, I asked Richard to
do nothing at all; then at least there would be a possibility that because
he was not himself thinking about standing, the ideo-motor action would
not occur.

But this didn't work, either. At the moment I moved Richard, he
became fixated on the idea of moving, with the result that he tensed his
neck, tightened in his chest and back, and performed the action himself,
in spite of his own intention to remain sitting. When, after being asked
to do nothing, Richard then made a special effort not to move, he only
became further preoccupied with the very idea that triggered the action.
The preoccupation with "doing" makes Richard susceptible, at the most
subtle mental level, to the very pattern of tension that we are trying to
prevent.

How, then, is it possible to break free of the associational process that
triggers the action? First, it is necessary for Richard to make a firm decision to do nothing, while allowing me to move him vicariously. He must,
in other words, exercise his capacity to stop, or to "inhibit," when the
impulse to act comes to him. He must then allow me to vicariously perform a series of movements that result in the desired end, in this way
experiencing a new way of performing the action without actually being
triggered into the old habitual pattern.

In order to succeed in this process, it is necessary to break the action down for Richard into discrete steps that do not associate with the finished act. For instance, the act of getting out of a chair can be broken down into the act of (1) hinging forward at the hips until the weight is over one's feet, and (2) straightening one's legs to rise onto one's feet. If Richard focuses entirely on the first step in this sequence, this provides a focus which distracts him from the idea of standing and avoids any association with the goal, or idea, of the finished act. Taken one step at a time, the finished act of standing can then be achieved without having thought of the end at all.

This process, however, is by no means simple to implement. At first, Richard invariably associates coming forward from the hips with his habitual reaction of standing. In spite of himself, he becomes concerned with results and tries to "get it right"—and he ends up "helping" and performing the entire act habitually. In spite of his belief that he can control what he's doing, he is getting the "idea" to do the action and is in fact performing it as he has always done it. It is necessary to get Richard not to think about the idea of performing the unwanted action by positively focusing his attention elsewhere. In this way, Richard's attention is diverted from the idea of standing, and it gives him in its place a more constructive focal point of attention.

This process entails a new focus on the part of the student attempting to master the principles of conscious awareness and control. Under normal circumstances, the person who is learning a new skill relies on a kind of faith that he can do what he wants to do, simply by trying various options until he hits on the right one. The student may attempt to relax, or try out a number of different ways of moving, but this approach inevitably invokes the subconscious operation of the muscular system, since, as we've seen, any action, however performed, brings into play the ideo-motor response. By focusing entirely on the component steps, however, the student is now able to circumvent the subconscious working of the system, and in this way he can reconstruct the activity in a more conscious, rational way. He will then be able to achieve the goal by relying entirely on the intermediate steps toward that goal without having to be continually fixated on the goal. He will become less concerned to do the action "correctly," and because of this, he will be able to pay more attention to the process that will actually result in that goal.

When Richard has mastered the first step—that is, learned to come forward from the hips without associating that movement with the act of standing—he is then ready to go on to the second step, adhering to the same principle, until he has completed the act of standing without associating the component steps with the habitual act of standing. Usually this experience is self-reinforcing: he finds that he is able to achieve his goal without being directly concerned with it. The process, in other words, becomes more interesting to him than the "end" for which he is working, and he thus learns to focus entirely on the means to his end without bringing into play the habitual act.

Once this step is mastered, it is then necessary for Richard to learn how to perform coordinated actions on his own. By allowing me to move him, and by then focusing on an intermediate action not related to standing, Richard has learned to avoid the idea of standing. As long as he maintained the lengthened condition and remained calm enough that he could successfully allow me to move him without succumbing to the temptation to make the movement himself, the old pattern could be avoided. When Richard attempts the same procedure *without* my help, however, the problem is far more complex. Now he has to perform the action himself, and how can he stand without thinking of standing?

When, for instance, Richard begins to come forward in the chair, he knows only one way of performing such a movement: as a preparation for standing. In spite of his best intentions, he will invariably begin the movement by tightening in the neck, pulling the head back, and bracing in the legs in anticipation of standing up—exactly the pattern he wants to avoid. When he then tries to alter this, he will do so not by stopping but by trying something else, which means that he will tighten in preparation to move, just as before, except that in addition to this he will superimpose other harmful movements over the original one.

This explains the problem Richard faces in attempting this procedure on his own. In performing actions, we are largely aware of our power to voluntarily control our own movements. Our usual assumption, in making such movements, is that if there is a problem, we can do something to correct that problem. Having experienced the condition he wants, Richard therefore assumes that he can achieve the desired condition by voluntarily reproducing it. But this, as we've seen, is a fallacy. In this case, the desired condition is the result not of performing a positive action, but of preventing one. When Richard attempts to reproduce the action, he is bringing into play the very thing he is attempting to avoid, and so there is no alternative but for the muscles to tighten as they always have as part of the habitual pattern of activity.

This problem is compounded by Richard's enthusiasm to succeed. The undesirable action happens precisely because Richard has the idea to do something, and it is the refusal to engage in the normal voluntary action that is therefore the key to success. When Richard tries to reproduce this action, however, he is not only failing to prevent the harmful pattern, but positively reproducing it, and every successive attempt is therefore part of the problem, not the solution. His desire to do the right action, then, only complicates the problem, because it means that, without taking the time to stop and think, he will blindly try to get the action right and mechanically repeat the old harmful set of habits.

In order to counteract this tendency, it is necessary, first, for Richard to decide that he mustn't act too quickly. Taking the time to think out the new action, he must then get the experience of doing the movement in an entirely new way, as the basis for counteracting the old subconscious pattern. Since coming forward in the chair is preparatory to standing, he must not only refuse to stand, but he must be prepared to perform an action that is, for all intents and purposes, entirely different than the action he has always made. In this way, he can avoid the harmful pattern of tension, precisely by avoiding the action with which it is associated.

Discovering how to make such a new action, however, requires discipline and practice. By learning new and unfamiliar actions, Richard must then learn to maintain the desired physical conditions and to focus on the necessary component steps of the process. He must be impressed with the importance of consciously thinking out each step in the process, taking each one in turn. The entire procedure requires a constant effort to stop and, in so doing, to prevent the ideo-motor pathway from operating. In this way, the action is reconstructed by shifting the focus away from the old pathway and into a new one.

In concrete terms, this means that the improvement in physical coordination makes possible an increased awareness and control over the ideo-motor response and, with it, an improved functioning. The tension in the neck and torso is part of a total response, a pathway of activity that is more or less unconscious. By restoring the working of the muscular system, and by then breaking apart the constellation of habits during the act itself, it is possible, for the first time, to find alternatives to the usual pattern of activity, to perform actions without the usual tensions and constrictions, and to interfere less with the natural reflex activity. This permits a normal condition of vitality and muscular tone, a coordinated working of parts, and a more natural breathing. In short, it makes it possible to circumvent the harmful influence of the ideo-motor pattern itself.

Performing actions in this way also provides the basis for thinking out consciously how to achieve ends that are normally pursued unconsciously. The ideo-motor response, as we've seen all along, is designed to work automatically, making it possible to achieve ends without thinking about the specifics of how the body achieves those results. Over the life span we develop a repertoire of extremely skilled actions that become stereotyped and highly ingrained. Precisely because these actions are so ingrained as habit, however, they impede the conscious performance of action. By deliberately examining our stereotyped actions, the physical and mental associations are broken down, the force of habit is weakened, and the ability to consciously think out actions—and to achieve the ends to which these actions are oriented—is developed and strengthened.

These changes now make it possible for Richard to perceive the role of his own actions in contributing to his back problem. Let's say that, after asking Richard to do nothing, I tell him that I would now like to stand him onto his feet. Earlier, when I moved Richard, he was unable to perceive whether he reacted harmfully to my suggestion; his entire system was triggered harmfully into action, without any consciousness on his part. The previous changes, however, have made it possible for Richard to perceive when he harmfully tenses himself during activity, and this enables him, for the first time, to begin to prevent the ideo-motor pattern itself. At the moment I bring Richard forward in the chair to stand, he will begin, unconsciously, to tighten in the neck, chest, and torso, and to impulsively stand up in anticipation of the action I have suggested to him. But because he has now experienced what it is like to lengthen, he can now begin to kinesthetically perceive how this activity—the entire pattern of unconscious tension—begins as a response pattern. This sensation at first will be vague, but he will observe with increasing clarity that, at a deeper layer, he is unconsciously tightening throughout the neck and torso, and thereby interfering with the entire supportive function of the spine and the muscular system.

This activity is now—at least to some extent—accessible to study and, therefore, to conscious prevention. On previous occasions, whenever I had moved Richard, the reaction had occurred so quickly, and the interference with the muscular system was so unconscious and ingrained, that there seemed little that either he or I could do about it. But with the adjustments and general improvements that our previous efforts have brought about, it is now possible for Richard to feel this pattern of response as it occurs. When I bring him forward and suggest the movement of standing, I can now point out the pattern and confront Richard with the reaction just as it begins. The next time I bring him forward in the chair, Richard can prevent the response and, by focusing on the process rather than on the end result, literally diffuse its impulse and release the tension pattern as it begins. Instead of tightening, he can now stop and, by recognizing the tendency to react automatically, release the tension as it begins in the neck, back, and chest. I can then bring Richard forward and onto his feet, without the usual tension and muscular interference.

Confronting the response in this way makes it possible to reveal and isolate the ideo-motor response and its interference with the body. We observed earlier that the pattern of tension was interfering with the reflex working of the postural mechanism by causing rigidity and collapse in the muscular system. Because the tension has been weakened, the internal support of the postural system is allowed to work, automatically supporting the chest and resulting in a release of chronic rigidity in the rib cage and chest, as well as an increased length and support through the torso. As the habitual muscular tension diminishes, parts of the chest that had been chronically tense regain mobility, and the body, which had been shortened because of the habitual interference, regains support and lightness. It is then possible to move Richard in and out of the chair, giving him the experience of length and flexibility while performing movements which he had previously performed in a strained and harmful manner.

This general change also influences Richard's particular symptom. Because the working of his lower back was dependent on the general working of the postural system, restoring the working of this system improves the condition of his back by reducing the shortening and arching of the lower back and strengthening the supporting function of the muscles of the back and trunk. In short, the specific condition of tension is improved upon by preventing the general pattern of misuse that had interfered with the working of the entire muscular system.

We can now begin to link the symptoms we initially observed to the problem of ideo-motor action. We observed, earlier, the pattern of tension that occurs during a simple action. This tension was linked, in turn, with an interference in the natural reflexive working of the postural system—rigidity and collapse that interfere with the normal functioning of the system. We then saw that this tension pattern is triggered by ideas during activity, and that this pathway of activity is the means by which normal action is produced. This showed that the tension pattern was neither physical nor mental, but was part of a pathway of activity in which ideas and tension occurred simultaneously in the context of a total response pattern.

Now that we have improved the working of the postural system, and then observed how the ideo-motor response interferes with this system, we can see how the total pathway of activity comes into play and reactivates the pattern of interference in the postural system. The problem, then, isn't the tension pattern *per se,* or the harmful physical condition it has caused, but the underlying activity that creates this condition. Until now these reactions were invisible, but now that they can be perceived, it is clear that underlying the physical problem is a pattern of activity linked to the ideo-motor pattern.

This represents a clear instance of the relation of ideo-motor action to physical functioning. Because we can improve upon the specific problem by removing the larger pattern of physical interference that has interfered with normal functioning, it is easy to be content with making the physical changes which bring about an improvement in this general condition. However, when we observe how the physical interference recurs even when the body is restored, then we are forced to recognize that the underlying cause—and the ultimate problem to be solved—is the pattern of ideo-motor action in which the entire system is brought into play as one pathway of response. What appeared to be a physical symptom, then, is traceable to a far deeper and more complex problem—the pattern of ideo-motor action in which ideas and motor activity function as one pathway.

To give another example, take the case of a computer user, whom we'll call Jane, who suffers from chronically tightened shoulders caused by prolonged periods of work at the keyboard. As we saw, it may not initially be clear that Jane's shoulder problem is connected with tensions produced while typing. But after making various adjustments, it becomes clear that her problem is in fact related to the way she is typing, and that her shoulder—once the system has been restored to its natural lengthened state—can function more normally in the context of this improved general condition. Observe, however, what happens once Jane is asked, while sitting at her desk, to raise the arm to the keyboard. At the moment she does so she stiffens the neck and back muscles, and the shoulder, which a moment ago had been functioning normally, will again be found to be stiffened. Even after I make repeated adjustments, and again restore the normal condition of the shoulder, the harmful condition will again reappear once she has the idea to type. But if, in contrast, she is able to notice this response and, while maintaining the improved condition, she allows me to raise her arm for her so that she can experience a more coordinated way of using the arm while preventing the interference, the harmful condition of the shoulder does not reappear. As long as she does not interfere with this new condition, she can type without experiencing the harmful condition of tension in the shoulder.

As in Richard's case, Jane's problem can now be seen in its proper relation to the underlying activity and the way in which that activity is subconsciously triggered by the idea of typing. The condition of the shoulder was symptomatic of a larger pattern of tension that interfered with the system. But we can now see that the problem was caused not by a harmful pattern of movement, nor by the chronic interference with the muscular system associated with this tension, but by its link with the pattern of activity that governs all of her voluntary actions. We can identify and improve upon the harmful condition in the body, but the pattern continues to be triggered as a total pathway of activity, and until we uncover this pathway and prevent it, the problem cannot be solved.

The same principle applies to various general problems in functioning. If, for instance, breathing is impaired by tightness in the ribs or by a generally collapsed condition, this problem cannot be addressed adequately simply by performing breathing exercises or by freeing the ribs—even if this is done during activity by trying to increase thoracic capacity while moving or speaking. The reason for this is, once activity resumes, the harmful pattern of interference will dominate any specific attempts to control or improve breathing. It is important, in such a case, to address the entire activation of the mechanism, and in so doing to stop the total pattern of interference that is at the root of the physical condition and which is undermining the general conditions of vitality and functioning that are associated with breathing.

We have now traced our initial physical symptom full circle to its relation to the subconscious pattern of activity. We first observed the pattern of tension, which we then saw was connected with the chronic interference in the postural system. We then observed the pattern of ideo-motor activity and could see that the very nature of the intention to act is at the root of this interference. In virtually every action Richard performed he had a tendency to interfere with this underlying system, and the tendency was so habitual and ingrained that he was completely unaware of it.

Although it was not immediately apparent, then, this ideo-motor activity is connected with—and ultimately at the root of—the chronic interference in the working of the muscular system. When we spoke earlier of the interference with the postural system that resulted from the tension pattern, we saw that this bodily condition of shortening and chronic rigidity needed to be rectified in order to restore the proper working of the body. But now that we have restored the system and observed the ideo-motor pattern and how it works, we can see that it is the pattern of action itself that impairs this system.

Even more significant is the fact that the problem can be ultimately linked to the mechanism by which Richard performs virtually all his actions. If when Richard consciously refrained from making harmful actions, he could not control this pattern of activity, then consider how powerful an influence it must be in all his voluntary actions, where the temptation to act is far stronger than in the artificial environment provided by a teacher examining his actions. Richard's pattern of activity might appear to be an aberration from normal conscious action, but it is the means by which he performs virtually all normal voluntary action during the course of his daily life.

Identifying this harmful underlying pattern of activity is crucial to clearly conceiving the cause of the problem we originally observed. I said, at the beginning of this book, that particular problems have emerged that cannot be adequately addressed through existing fields. As long as we can achieve adequate results by treating or making adjustments to the body or developing methods of bodywork that address physical holdings and tensions, we are justified in employing such methods as a means of solving these problems. But because the bodily condition or tension is in fact perpetuated by the pattern of activity, then it is necessary, ultimately, to address not the bodily condition, but the pattern of activity itself, and no method of bodywork or treatment can make such a result possible. If we accurately observe how the body works and how it is interfered with as a physical system, then we are led inexorably to a concept of activity in which mind and body are seen to function as one unified pathway of activity. Methods for relaxation or treating bodily conditions cannot address a problem that requires, ultimately, that we gain conscious awareness and control of our actions.

The role of ideo-motor action in contributing to the immediate cause of the problem also provides a clue as to the origins of the problem. Earlier, we observed that in civilized life the postural system in humans is very easily thrown out of adjustment, and identified this as a fundamental cause of the tendency to acquire faulty use. But by itself, the postural mechanism will tend to work correctly when not interfered with; it is the ideo-motor function that perpetuates the interference in this system. This suggests that, over time, it is the harmful actions associated with the ideo-motor mechanism, and not the faulty working of the postural system, that caused the problem to begin with. Through repeated faulty action, the postural system is increasingly compromised until, finally, specific parts of the system cannot work properly, and symptoms develop. In this sense, the original problem cannot be blamed on the failure of the postural mechanism itself, but on the harmful action associated with it.

Observing the connection of specific problems to activity, however, is not always self-evident. If, as we saw in Richard's case, the chest was tense and shortened, then when he moved it would be difficult to perceive how the ideo-motor response itself could be the cause of such a condition. When this chronic condition was reduced by restoring the normal working of his system, it was then possible to perceive that the tension occurs as part of the actual pathway of activity. With the condition thus improved, it was then possible to see that at the moment that he made an action Richard collapsed and shortened in the chest, that the tension in the chest occurred as part of an actual pathway of activity, and that this pathway of activity was therefore the cause of the interference in the system.

In a general sense, then, it is easy to observe the pattern of ideo-motor action as a basic mechanism of action. But it is far more difficult to perceive the direct influence of the ideo-motor pattern on the interference in his postural system in particular activities. This required, first, that the physical system be restored to such an extent that under a teacher's guidance Richard could perform actions without grossly interfering with the postural system and, second, that Richard could begin to kinesthetically perceive the pattern of tension as it occurs. This made it possible, in turn, to improve further how the system is working, and provided the basis for identifying the harmful pattern of activity and its direct role in contributing to the symptom.

CHAPTER FIVE

Reaction and the Problem of Stress

Reaction and Stress

We have now outlined the basic features of the problem that we originally set out to understand. Following our initial observations of a harmful pattern of tension, we then saw that motor acts are linked with ideas
as one pathway. Richard's physical symptoms were caused, ultimately,
by what he was himself doing in action.

But there are several questions still unanswered. So far we have identified the pattern of tension, and we know that it is harmful because it
interferes with the body's innate design. Once we linked the harmful
pattern of tension with ideas, it became clear that the problem was not
limited to the impaired working of the muscular system, but involved a
total pattern of action that was itself wrong. But what does it mean to
say that the pattern of ideo-motor action is working incorrectly? If the
ideo-motor function is imbalanced, does this involve a mental as well as
a physical imbalance? And why does this function become imbalanced
to begin with?

This will be the subject of the next several sections. In the study of
stress, the usual approaches identify a harmful physical condition that,
based on research on the physiology of stress, is linked with stressors or
outside influences which have brought about this harmful condition.
Methods are then applied in order to reduce the condition of stress, often
based on the ability to learn new responses by thinking differently, altering one's mental attitude, and practicing relaxation techniques. In spite
of this observed connection of mental states with physiological responses,
however, such approaches assume that the physical problem is caused by
mental or emotional responses, and thus separate mind and body in the
very act of insisting on unity. When we look further at the unified pattern of action that we have now identified and at the process of solving

it, a new mental and physical dimension in the analysis of stress becomes apparent, and it becomes possible to conceive of stress in a more complete way.

Let's return to Richard and his tendency to stand uncontrollably onto his feet when he is sitting and is given the idea of standing. The reason for this uncontrolled action, of course, is already familiar to us. Subconsciously I have given Richard the idea of standing, and his pattern of tension, which indicates a tendency to respond to ideas, is invoked when I begin to move him. He is triggered into the action against his will. But this action is, as we also have said, a response we don't want; it is an uncontrolled reaction. When a door is slammed unexpectedly, we are meant to be startled; such an instinctive reaction, or protective response, is appropriate to the situation and is in this sense "meant" to happen. But in Richard's case, we haven't slammed a door or startled him in any way. In fact, we haven't done anything that would elicit an involuntary or instinctive reaction. Suggesting the act of standing is not a sufficient stimulus to produce an involuntary response.

We saw earlier that this reaction was caused by a distortion, or overexcitation, of the ideo-motor pattern—a tendency to short-circuit into action, to perform actions too readily when presented with an idea, or stimulus, to do something. This tendency, we said, represents a problem not simply in the working of the body but in the entire mental and physical pathway of activity. We also observed that because such a reaction is viewed as a bodily function, it is not regarded as particularly significant—nothing more than a harmless tendency, not unlike that found in elderly people, to become startled when surprised or under pressure. In the present case, however, it is an impeding factor in Richard's progress, since it is impossible for him to prevent the tension pattern as long as he is continuing to jump too readily into activity.

How, then, is it possible to prevent Richard's response? Richard recognizes that he is in a worked-up state, and he knows that he needs to somehow become more calm. He attributes his condition to the fact that he is worried or anxious, and he believes that this emotional attitude causes him to be physically tense. He is able, by directly attempting to relax his physical state or by changing his mental attitude, to control specific muscles. But interestingly, he continues to overreact when presented with a simple task such as rising from a sitting position. While attempting to maintain a relaxed condition, his effort to focus on not doing the action only intensifies his preoccupation with the action itself, and he continues to react as before. The problem, if it is to be solved, must address not simply his body but the total pathway of action and reaction.

I discussed earlier several stages involved in changing the reaction. First, I identified the tensions in the back of the neck, the lower back, shoulders, and legs. By making various adjustments and encouraging the tensions to release, the body becomes springier, and the torso begins to lighten and become less constricted. It is clear, however, that Richard will begin to constrict and strain again once he goes into movement, so it is necessary to remind him to slow down and not to make any movement himself. By breaking the movement down into discrete components, we are able to reconstruct actions by focusing on the means and not the end. Step by step, the tensions will begin to release until there is an increasing sense of mobility through the body. As the state of tension through the body diminishes, the harmful pattern of motor activity is removed, and the tendency to jump into activity when I move him is reduced.

With each session, Richard's condition improves and calms down until, at a certain point, the entire state calms down. The breathing becomes freer, and the overactive pattern of tension dissipates. The reduced state of physical activity is accompanied by a change in mental state as well. He doesn't seem as preoccupied or worried as before. He becomes more alert and more deliberate in his learning process, the whole system calms down, and the tendency to jump into activity—the reaction itself—begins to dissipate.

This calming down is accompanied also by an alteration in emotional state. Richard's state of tension is associated with an emotional condition of stress and worry. This state is particularly noticeable in his face, which shows a strained and preoccupied look, and in the preoccupied and distracted look in his eyes. As Richard calms down, however, his mental attitude improves, his face and eyes become more animated, his mood improves, and he becomes more mentally alert. In short, his change in reaction and physical condition is accompanied by a dissipation of worry and emotional preoccupation.

These changes demonstrate the underlying significance of the reaction we have observed from the outset. Until now I've talked about the connection between ideas and motor acts. In observing the tension pattern connected with this pattern of ideo-motor action, we saw that Richard's activities were too easily triggered, but since my intention was to examine the connection between the two, we did not make any particular value judgment as to whether it was unhealthy or not. But Richard was in an overwrought state, and as that state improves, there is an overall decrease in tension and muscular activity. The entire system quiets down and becomes calm, the breathing becomes freer, and the nervous reactions seem to shut off. It is as if until the release throughout Richard's body was brought about, the entire system was charged with physical and mental energy, and that energy is now able to quiet down. The tension pattern being triggered into activity is like an underlying short circuit that comes into play too readily, and it will increasingly weaken in intensity until, finally, the entire system returns to a truly calm condition, and the triggered reaction disappears entirely.

The reaction, then, was symptomatic of a fundamental problem that, until now, was not apparent. It was not, simply, that Richard's pattern of action was harmful to the working of the body. The reactive pattern is indicative of what is, in effect, a disturbed condition of the entire system. To the casual observer, this pattern might not appear to be a serious problem. Apart from the fact that he is slightly nervous and ill at ease, there appears to be nothing wrong with Richard. But underlying his overt reactions is a subtle but distinctly noticeable state of muscular and nervous excitement and mental preoccupation. Instead of a balanced, relaxed way of moving and doing things, there is a level of tension and effort and distortion in doing that implies a wrong working of Richard's muscular system. Instead of a calm and balanced way of responding to the stimulus to do something, his tendency to respond too quickly and to have no control over his responses implies an unhealthy level of reactivity in behavior. And instead of an alert, conscious attitude, there is a mental overinvolvement, almost a mentally distracted quality. In short, the pattern of tensions we initially observed is really one aspect of a disturbance, an imbalanced operation, of the entire behavioral machinery.

The full significance of the ideo-motor pathway and its excitability in action, then, is not clear until we link it with the disturbed condition that is now apparent in Richard. Because it was necessary to show how mind and body work as a total, unified mechanism, I focused, in the first few chapters, specifically on the mental and physical pathway of activity. But remember that what led us to look at this mechanism to begin with was a problem, and we did not identify what that problem was. In the normal ideo-motor response, it should not be possible to trigger someone into activity against his will, but Richard's condition represents an intensification of that ideo-motor response. As long as Richard is subconsciously preoccupied with that stimulus, he will continue to jump out of the chair, because that tension pattern represents a tendency to respond to an idea even when he has chosen not to. And this intensified response indicates a disturbed condition of the entire mechanism.

This shows how important this abnormal ideo-motor response really is. It constitutes not merely a wrong working of the body or an unwanted movement. It indicates a state of functioning of the mind and body that is, to put it simply, associated with stress and disturbance. As I will show in a moment, if we want to fully understand the problem of stress, we must recognize the significance of the pattern of ideo-motor action and its association with disturbance in daily living. The wrong working of the ideo-motor mechanism is in fact a wrong reaction that is directly associated with, and a fundamental cause of, stress; no alteration in one's physical condition can completely restore a healthy and calm condition in living when this problem is present.

This connection between the tension pattern and the intensified ideo-motor response also explains, at least in part, why the problem has developed. The wrong working of the body is associated with a tendency for the pathway of activity to erupt into activity too easily, for subconscious mental associations to short-circuit into motor acts. Conversely, when the physical system is in balance, this tends to restore the pattern of reaction to the normal state, and the body is no longer susceptible to being triggered into activity. In short, the pattern of tension we've observed, and which has been so difficult to solve because it occurs as a reaction, is nothing less than a breakdown, or a disintegration, of the normal ideo-motor response. The ideo-motor mechanism—the muscular system as it works in conjunction with thought processes to produce motor activity—has become overly stimulated to the point that the controls in action have broken down, and Richard has lost full command over his actions. And this loss of control, in turn, is accompanied by an increased overall state of excitability, or stress.

Perceiving this connection also gives us a clue as to how the pattern developed. Once there is an increase in tension in the system, the original intact ideo-motor pathway becomes overstimulated. Over time, normal ideo-motor action becomes increasingly susceptible to discharge, and actions become uncontrolled, agitated, and compulsive. If you observe small children, you will never see actions of this sort. Children do, of course, experience irritability and other mood changes that accompany different needs and emotional frustrations. But the child's natural functional state is calm and free from the tense and overwrought condition so characteristic of adults. Action, except when the child is under the influence of unusually strong emotional states, is calm and deliberate—which is only to say that the mechanism of action is intact at birth. Under the influence of constant misuse, however, the pathway of activity becomes increasingly excited and there is a loss of inhibitory control and calmness in action until, with time, the pattern of tension and reaction becomes the norm.

The reactive condition, then, signifies a breakdown in the working of the ideo-motor pathway. As that condition worsens, it becomes increasingly associated with loss of control and an associated condition of stress and disturbance. When the normal working of this mechanism is restored, the tendency to react dissipates and the entire system calms down. By restoring the normal pathway of activity, the disturbance associated with the disintegration in the pathway of ideo-motor activity is removed.

We have now traced the original observation of a pattern of tension to a problem of reaction that is associated with disturbance. Underlying this pattern of response is a condition of stress that is directly associated with the wrong working of this mechanism and which can be corrected only by restoring its normal working. The full meaning of this unwanted reaction, then, is that it represents a disintegrated working of the ideomotor pattern that is associated with a condition of disturbance, or stress. And the only way to restore the calm state is to restore the mechanism to a balanced state.

Let me give another example in order to make this clearer—the case of a woman who suffered from tension in the forearms while typing. When I first observed Susan, it was clear that she was an active, energetic person. Although she spent many hours at a computer, she was in good health, and the physical pain she complained of did not seem to be associated with an unusual degree of constriction or collapse in her muscular system. And yet when I asked her to perform some simple movements, it at once became clear that she was in fact in a high state of tension and had virtually no control over her actions. For instance, when I asked her to remain sitting while I stood her up, she was so quick to jump out of the chair that there did not even seem any point in telling her not to. In fact, once she understood that I intended to stand her up, she no longer seemed to fully sit in the chair: she was tensed and poised on the edge of her seat before I had even begun to move her. When I explained to her that the whole point of my moving her this way was to give her a chance to calm down and to use less muscular effort, she still jumped out of the chair at my slightest suggestion, without even realizing she was doing so.

As with Richard, Susan is reactive—so much so that when I move her she is almost startled into action. But in contrast to Richard, we can recognize instantly that there is something wrong: she is so overly stimulated, and her mental state so distracted, that we know instantly there is a problem. But exactly what kind of problem is it? We are likely to say, in her case, that her condition is emotional, and in fact it is essential to address her emotional state so that she will feel more comfortable and be in a more receptive state.

But if we want to help Susan, we must address her reactive tendency as well, and in this sense her problem, though different in degree, is the same as Richard's. Her tendency, at work, has been to perform actions

so quickly and under such constant pressure that she is virtually inca-
pable, having now worked in this way for many years, of performing
the action of typing except in a rushed and agitated way. The reason for
this imbalanced activity is that the inhibitory control that is inherent in
Susan's normal ideo-motor response has disintegrated. In order to control her reaction, it is necessary to restore the normal working of the mechanism by lowering the level of muscular energy, and then by raising her
consciousness in action so that she can again control her actions and restore
a normal level of energy. The pattern will then no longer be intensified
in its operation, and she will regain the capacity to act calmly and deliberately.

Susan's case, though, is more complicated than Richard's. On the one
hand, she is in such a state of physical tension that it is essential, as a first
step, to bring about a healthier condition of muscle activity. On the other
hand, her emotional state demands that she be given a sensitive and supportive environment that encourages her to feel at ease, to think with
more clarity, and to calm down. In fact, Susan's case may require outside emotional work—a subject that I will address in a moment. But as
with Richard, the level of her reaction is itself a problem that is not, in
essence, emotional but related to activity. Although her reactive tendency appears to be symptomatic of an emotional state, it is in fact indicative of a breakdown in motor function. When the associated condition
of the muscular system is improved, this change will increasingly restore
the natural calm function of the whole mechanism and create a more
balanced mental and physical state.

Susan's tendency to react when performing basic everyday actions is a
major source of stress in her life. The normal working of the ideo-motor
function has broken down, leading to a disturbed condition over which
she has little control. As in Richard's case, the wrong working of the ideo-
motor action constitutes a harmful level of reaction that is directly associated with, and a fundamental cause of, stress. By observing the reaction
associated with the ideo-motor pathway of activity, it is possible to identify this condition not as a vague response to outside stressors but as a
direct result of the level of functioning of her own system in activity. If
Richard and Susan want to solve their problem, they must gain control

over their own reactions, and this can happen only if they become aware of and gain control over the actions that are associated with reaction.

It is important to remember, though (to return to Richard's case), that Richard has no way of seeing any of this. He is not aware of his ideo-motor function, how it works or what might be wrong with it, or that the deterioration in its working is associated with disturbance. As outside observers, we have the benefit of objectively "testing" Richard's actions and observing the connection between his muscular action and the ideas that trigger them—and even then, it is not easy to detect these problems. But it is virtually impossible for Richard to subjectively perceive the pattern of ideo-motor action in himself, the harmful tension pattern that has developed, or the associated level of reaction. He experiences symptoms, but he does not know where they come from.

This has important implications for the study of stress and the mind/body area generally. If Richard experiences symptoms of tension or stress at work, he assumes they come from outside sources. When, therefore, he practices a relaxation technique or method for reducing stress, he feels that, when he reduces his symptoms of stress, he is addressing the problem. But the results he achieves in this way will not address the disturbance associated with his own action and reaction, which will remain essentially unchanged. In fact, he doesn't really even know he is in a disturbed condition. Identifying the symptom with the problem, he believes that when he alleviates these symptoms, he *is* solving the problem. But the underlying cause of these symptoms does not lie outside himself, but in the working of his own organism.

This is true of virtually everyone who suffers from everyday stress. Not being aware of the mechanism as a unified whole, and of the disturbance that is associated with its wrong, reactive working, the average person perceives symptoms as emanating from outside, or emotional, sources. The assumption is then made that by treating symptoms the problem will be solved. But the true source of this type of stress is the harmful working of the ideo-motor mechanism, which is virtually impossible to subjectively perceive and therefore will not be identifiable as the cause of the problem. If one does notice one's own harmful condition of strain or "nerves," or is medically and psychologically evaluated and found to be in a harmful condition, these qualities are usually characterized as symptomatic of outside stress or manifestations of emotional problems, not as an indication of something wrong in the working of the organism itself.

The same is true with Susan. In her case, of course, we know there is a problem: her nervous condition is easily identifiable. Again, however, we make the same mistake as we did in Richard's case—namely, we overlook the association of her disturbance with the breakdown of the ideo-motor mechanism, and so fail to perceive the full significance of the condition. The difference is that because Richard appears to be normal, we assume the stress emanates from outside him, whereas in Susan's case, it is clear that her condition is abnormal. But because we vaguely attribute this condition to emotions or to a response to outside stressors, we overlook the real cause in Susan's case in the same way as we did in Richard's.

In Susan's case, there are, as I said earlier, crucial emotional factors that must be addressed. But direct attempts to reduce the condition of stress or to understand underlying emotional causes do not alter the reactive tendency in action that is associated with stress. The emotional aspect of her problem is associated with her own reactions, and that is why she can't solve her problem by trying to reduce the stress or its emotional components directly. The emotional state is connected with the pattern of response, and the only way for her to solve her problem is to restore the pattern to its normal working.

It is interesting to note that, in contrast to Richard, Susan is more likely to be aware of her problem, whose manifestations are almost as obvious to her as to an outside observer. But she is not aware of the actual pattern of reaction of which it is a part. Part of the reason for this, as we've seen, is that the ideo-motor pathway is meant to work subconsciously; it is virtually impossible for her to detect this activity in herself. But even if this tendency is pointed out to her, she still does not connect it with her nervous symptoms, which she perceives as a "condition" that has either physical or emotional causes. Only when she can begin to gain control over her own actions and perceives a corresponding change in her level of stress can she see that her level of stress is actually associated with her own tendency, in daily life, to react when performing actions.

The reactive working of the ideo-motor mechanism, then, is a fundamental and unrecognized problem that relates directly to action. I said at the introduction to this book that many of the current mind/body methods represent an attempt to solve a class of problems that have not been adequately addressed by medicine and psychology. Methods have been presented without clarifying what the problem is, offering relief based on the assumption that to do so is to tap into the potential of the mind to heal the body. But such methods not only fail to address the true relation of mind and body; they also fail to empower the individual to gain control over the harmful reactions that cause the problem. If, for instance, Richard is able to reduce the stress associated with work, he thinks that he is thereby gaining control over his stress response. But why does he respond to work in such a way to begin with, when another person in a similar situation does not feel any stress at all? Richard's very concept of stress presupposes not that he can gain control over the response but that he must recover from something he has little control over. In other words, it presupposes that the only solution available to him is to recover from the harmful condition, not to understand its causes and to prevent it in the first place.

When he is able to observe his own activity, however, Richard is able not only to reduce the condition of stress but actually to alter his usual response to the situation that produces it. If disturbance is associated with one's own actions, then the only complete mind/body technique for removing stress is to gain control over these actions. Some techniques for reducing stress do in fact suggest ways of altering one's response to stressful situations, but such suggestions are not taken far enough and lack the crucial element of conscious control that is essential to achieving this goal.

We can now see why stress-reduction techniques fail to address fully the problem of stress. Symptoms of stress are associated, in daily activity, with a high level of reaction, and only by gaining a conscious awareness and control of this activity is it possible to reduce the disturbance associated with this activity, as well as to acquire an increasing ability to respond differently in situations that produce stress. The real problem in dealing with stress is to understand reaction, its various forms and its causes, and to empower the individual to address reaction in living by gaining a practical understanding of the mental and physical mechanism of action and reaction.

But why, if reaction is so critical, has its role in stress been overlooked? There are several reasons. First, I said earlier that when we observe reaction in its various forms, it is seen as a symptom of emotional and external factors and so has not been taken seriously in and of itself. This could not be otherwise, until the experience of what it is like to gain control over reactions makes it possible to perceive that, as in Richard's case, the disturbed condition is related to reaction itself, and that these reactions cannot be corrected through relaxation or other methods.

Second, in its most extreme forms, reaction is a symptom of mental illness and disturbance, as in the case of individuals who have suffered severe abuse or other forms of emotional trauma. In such cases, the body is in a state of alarm, and the corresponding level of reaction is abnormally high due to purely emotional factors. Because psychology has proceeded largely from a study of pathology, such harmful levels of reaction have been associated with the physiology of post-traumatic stress disorder and other forms of emotional stress. Reaction itself is then viewed as a symptom of this condition, and not in its relation to motor activity.

Third, it was impossible to discover how to achieve a calm and balanced state without first making other discoveries. The first, we saw, was how the physical mechanism was working wrongly and what was involved in restoring its balance. Based on this first step, it was then possible to see how muscular activity linked with ideas in one continuous pathway. This in turn made it possible to see that when this mechanism was working wrongly, it was associated with harmful reactions that are linked with stress. The discovery of a physical mechanism also made it possible to actually calm the system down and in so doing provided the key to solving the problem of reaction.

In short, a series of discoveries need to be made in order to see the full significance of reaction and its relation to stress. Without these discoveries, we can only perceive reaction as a bodily event and therefore dismiss it as symptomatic of "emotional" causes—an assumption that, as

I said earlier, is based on the intellectual prejudice that places emotional and mental factors in a higher category than physical ones and that accordingly regards physical reaction and bodily states as a manifestation of emotional and mental causes. The types of reaction we have observed in Richard and Susan are not symptomatic of mental causes but are associated with imbalanced and unconscious ideo-motor activity that must be brought under conscious control.

The types of reaction we have observed in Richard and Susan, however, take various other forms. The contrast between Richard and Susan, for instance, illustrates the extent to which the ideo-motor function can break down. In some cases, the tension pattern is not associated with an overtly overactive state. Some people, for instance, are physically tense, and yet they are, at the same time, calm in demeanor. They are not easily "triggered" into activity and are able to perform simple actions in a deliberate, controlled manner. In Richard and Susan the functioning of the ideo-motor mechanism has become overly stimulated to the point that the ability to remain calm in action is lost, leading eventually to outright loss of control. In Susan this deterioration had developed to such a point that she was in an emotionally disturbed state and had lost virtually all control in certain activities.

In cases where this breakdown or deterioration is fairly extreme, there is a corresponding deterioration in the physical mechanism. The level of reaction, in other words, is directly related to a loss of motor control and tension and strain in the system, which in turn result in increasing malcoordination and physical disturbance. In cases where reaction becomes extreme, muscular strength is diminished with a corresponding lowering of health and vitality.

Reaction also takes qualitatively different forms. Margaret, an accomplished pianist, had spent many years playing and performing extensively. She complained of physical tension, but she was unaware of the connection of her muscular tension with her reactions, which took the form of a loss of motor control and jitteriness. The disintegration of the pathway of action was so complete that when I asked her to allow me to move her arms for her, she literally could not keep them still. In her case, the tension problems are directly connected with a reactive tendency that has developed largely in relation to piano playing, although she is mildly disturbed and agitated during speech and other activities as well. Although her reactive tendency is connected with a high degree of tension and discomfort while playing, this harmful tendency does not interfere with her high level of skill at the piano, which she achieved at the expense of a balanced and calm manner of performing actions.

Melissa came to me because of a back problem, but her problem took an entirely different form than the previous cases. She had been a housewife her whole life, and was compulsively efficient. She exhibited a marked loss of control in simple actions and a stooped, awkward way of bending and walking. Her main problem, however, was her mentally distracted condition. She was so accustomed to rushing and doing several things at once that it was as if she was not "all there"; her distracted state made it very difficult to reach her mentally, to get her to actually think in a new way and to hear a new idea. In addition to her agitated condition, her harmful reaction had resulted in a deterioration that could only be described as mental.

Another form of reaction in which mental preoccupation is the complicating factor is found in those who do highly intellectualized work. John, for instance, was a lawyer who was constantly called upon to analyze difficult documents. The many years he devoted to highly demanding intellectual work manifested as a form of mental preoccupation, a tendency to intellectualize even during physical activity. Within the context of his work, John was highly capable and alert, but he was remarkably unobservant in outside matters. In contrast, some people are mentally observant and alert in general matters, and yet compulsive in doing things. In this case the problem is not a mental preoccupation but, very simply, the intensity of the drive to do and achieve. This tendency is often found in people who are otherwise quite calm and capable; in fact, the compulsion is to some extent a function of their clarity and focus.

Another common form of reaction that must be mentioned is compulsiveness in speech. Speech, being closely connected with cognitive processes as well as communicating, is a powerful and sometimes addictive stimulus. Individuals who indulge in speech for many years without the discipline of speaking slowly or formulating ideas carefully often develop the tendency to speak too quickly, compulsively, or with a high degree of tension and excitability. Because speech involves the muscles of the neck, back, and torso, as well as the entire breathing mechanism, these tendencies can often impair breathing and interfere with general bodily poise, leading to a condition of outright tension and collapse.

In its mental form, reaction also manifests in the form of insomnia. When physical activity ceases, reaction tends to cease as well. But reaction that is associated with mental activities such as computer programming or writing tends to persist even during periods of rest. In this sense, insomnia is a disturbance not so much of sleep as of waking activity; insomnia, or the inability of the brain to switch over into sleep, is a manifestation of an imbalance in the mechanism not of sleep but of action.

Common to these various forms of reaction is the disintegration of the ideo-motor pathway; the various types of reaction listed above simply reflect the differences in mental and physical demands associated with different types of activities. In some cases the disturbance manifests in a "mental" form, as in cases where intellectual activity or constant worrying over details creates mental fixation or distraction; in other cases the physical aspect of the problem is more noticeable. But even apparently physical symptoms are connected with a tendency to react subconsciously; identifying the extent to which the normal pathway of activity has become disturbed is critical to removing the underlying interference. Once this connection of muscular tensions with increased reaction becomes discernable, it becomes equally evident that under the constant strain and pressure of modern civilized conditions, most adults are in a mildly disturbed state. With skill and experience in observation, it is not difficult to identify the extent to which someone has become overexcited or reactive, to perceive the level of tension and the degree of excitability in the muscular system, and to distinguish the different qualities of excitability or overstimulation that go hand in hand with the ideo-motor response.

The Psychology of Reaction

We have now begun to formulate a theory of stress based on the unified concept of mind and body that is the central theme of this book. By observing the continuity of mental associations and muscular tension in voluntary actions, and by then observing what was involved in changing this reaction, we have uncovered a fundamental and unrecognized problem that has to be addressed in order to deal with the problem of stress—the problem of reaction.

I want to turn now to the mind/body field itself and to try to place the problem of reaction in its proper context within that field. The mind/body field is very broad and borrows from a number of subjects addressing widely varying problems. Stress-reduction techniques focus primarily on reducing states of stress which are seen to be caused by various stressors. Other methods focus on the emotional causes of stress. Still other methods provide a means of producing a calm mental state. The underlying rationale for most of these approaches is that because mind and body are closely connected, therapeutic techniques for "harnessing" the power of the mind over the body can reverse the effects of stress. Yet among these various theories and therapeutic techniques, one finds virtually no mention of the problem of reaction, and therefore no mention of how to solve this problem. This means that we are faced not only with a new discovery but also the problem of assessing the validity of existing conceptions that operate without this discovery.

It could be argued that traditional methods do alter the level of reaction. But we know from the nature of reaction and how it operates as a total pattern of activity that therapeutic methods cannot solve a problem that requires awareness and control of voluntary action. Richard may make direct attempts at relaxation, release emotions associated with tensions, or increase mental awareness, but no matter how much he may feel relaxed and calmed down, once he engages in activity his reactions, as well as his muscular system, will return to their normally overactive state. Only an increased awareness of the ideo-motor pattern itself can possibly solve the problem, and this involves knowledge of how that mechanism works, observation of what has interfered with it, and conscious attention to its use in action. The view of mind and body as connected entities is simply inadequate to address a problem that is educational in nature, for the simple reason that such a view fails to address the problem of reaction itself and the disturbance associated with it. We must therefore arrive at a conception more appropriate to the unified function of reaction.

Let's look now at the problem of reaction and some of its special psychological characteristics in more detail. Earlier, we observed Richard in the everyday act of writing with a pen, and we observed that, like most people, he unnecessarily strained the muscles of his arm and hand once he began to write. After making adjustments in order to reduce the habitual level of tension, I then explained to him that because he tended to use too much tension in holding the pen, I would place the pen in his hand for him. When I brought the pen toward his hand, however, he began to stare at it and then, when I actually placed it in his hand, he impulsively reached for it, tightening his arm and hand and shoulder even when I asked him not to. When I again reminded him that I wanted him to do nothing, and instead to let me place the pen in his hand, he again stared at the pen, preoccupied with holding it, and again grabbed it as I placed it in his hand.

This, as we saw earlier, is a clear instance of ideo-motor action occurring as a reaction. The idea of writing, which is evoked by my asking Richard not to hold the pen and then by bringing the pen near his hand, issues into a motor act. A certain degree of muscular tension is of course required to perform this act, but if, as in Richard's case, the pathway is over-excited, then he will be too easily triggered into the action when I suggest it to him. This will result in a harmful reaction that, as we saw in the last chapter, is associated with disturbance.

Notice in particular the mental aspect of this reaction. We know that the action of taking the pen, which this time occurred clearly as a reaction, is a response to the subconscious idea of writing or taking hold of the pen. But Richard didn't simply have the idea to write or hold the pen. He first became fixated on, or mentally preoccupied with, the pen, and that mental fixation inevitably resulted in an uncontrolled reaction. Richard can't prevent the reaction because it begins with a mental or psychological preoccupation which triggers that particular pathway of activity. His response, in other words, is not simply a physical response to the idea of grabbing the pen, nor simply a finished act. It is a reaction that begins with a mental fixation, an intensified level of mental preoccupation, and this mental preoccupation results in an uncontrolled and reactive response.

This mental preoccupation explains why the unwanted reaction occurs. I said earlier that muscular activity is part of a pathway of ideas and motor activity. If, as we saw in the last section, this pathway is over-excited, then it will be associated with disturbance, giving it a significance that makes it important, not just physically, but to the study of stress as well. But remember that this reaction wasn't supposed to occur. If Richard's actions were balanced, the ideo-motor response wouldn't be triggered simply by placing the pen in his hand. His preoccupation with the pen indicates that he has become subconsciously distracted by, or fixated on, the stimulus, and this explains why the unwanted reaction takes place.

The action of taking the pen, then, is not simply caused by an idea that triggers a physical action and that, in turn, is associated with a harmful level of disturbance in the system. We must include, as part of our conception of the unified functioning of mind and body in action, a harmful mental state as well. Richard's pattern of response involves not only a physical set of tensions and an actual movement, but also a mental preoccupation, a mental overinvolvement, in performing the act—an involvement that is so strong that it overcomes even his conscious intentions. When the stimulus is presented, he can't help but be subconsciously and mentally preoccupied with it, and this response connotes an unhealthy subconscious preoccupation that triggers the action. The tension pattern, then, isn't simply a wrong use of the body during behavior; it isn't even just a response pattern. It is a cultivated and overactive tendency to get the idea to react, and to actually react, outside of his own control.

We can now conceive of the problem of reaction in terms which begin to do justice to its psychological complexity. We saw, earlier, how muscular tension is linked with ideas to produce action, and how this activity must be addressed in order to prevent the pattern of tension. This pathway of activity, we also saw, is overactive and therefore linked with disturbance. But the mental preoccupation explains a crucial aspect of what is wrong in Richard: it represents a complication of the subconscious pattern of associations in normal ideo-motor action and thus explains in psychological terms how ideo-motor action can become reactive.

This psychological component is crucial to understanding the problem of reaction. In the earlier chapters on ideo-motor action, we saw that action is based on ideas that trigger motor acts, and we then examined whether this mental component was truly significant in any way. If the problem, we asked, is really physical, then why is the mental component significant except insofar as it must be addressed in order to correct the physical problem? The answer was that the problem wasn't physical but was actually caused by a total pathway of action that must itself be addressed in order to prevent the harmful physical tension that caused the problem. But the problem is even more complex than that. The reactive working of the normal pattern of ideo-motor action represents a complication of the subconscious mental activity that triggers motor activity, and in this sense is fundamentally psychological. Once we perceive the problem of ideo-motor action as a harmful reaction that is caused by a complication of the subconscious factor in action, then we must acknowledge that the problem of harmful physical tension is rooted in a disturbance in the psychology of action itself.

This psychological component becomes clearer if we look at it from the point of view of the psychological aspect of reaction. Think, for instance, of the phenomenon of jumping when a door has been slammed. Clearly such a reaction is physical, since the startle pattern is a physical response to a stimulus. But the reaction is just as much mental—a perceptual responsiveness to the stimulus of the sound. The nature of Richard's problem, being a kind of reaction, is very much the same thing. It is difficult to characterize his actions as mental or physical, because they are a combination. The pattern of tension represents the physical action, the reaction itself. But the reaction wouldn't happen at all were it not for his receptivity to be stimulated and his tendency to become preoccupied subconsciously, which represent the mental aspect. The tension, then, corresponds to the physical reaction; the mental preoccupation corresponds to the stimulus, or the receptivity to be stimulated; and the two together constitute the entire act, the response. The psychology of Richard's problem, then, possesses many of the same elements as that of instinctive reaction.

But Richard's reaction is different than the instinctive reaction in the following sense. The response to danger is innate; it is a built-in protective response that, in many cases, is purely reflexive and unthinking. Richard's reaction, however, represents an imbalanced working of a normal voluntary function—a tendency to react when he should normally be calm, and a tendency to become mentally involved in the thing he is reacting to when he need not even care about it. We saw that when his mechanism was adjusted and the reaction slowed down, his action was more calm and balanced, and he ceased to be subconsciously fixated on the action when it was suggested to him. Richard's reaction, then, represents a "pathological" form of a normal function, and the psychological complication is a crucial aspect of this "pathology."

Richard's reaction, then, shouldn't be a reaction, and what makes it so is not just the physical tension, but also the psychological component. In the earlier discussion of ideo-motor action, we saw that the mental and physical elements corresponded to stimulus and response—the stimulus corresponding to the mental aspect, or idea, and the response corresponding to the action, or motor act. But consider again in more detail what this mental side means. In order to respond to a stimulus, we have to be receptive to inner or outer influences in such a way that we are able to respond. Having received the stimulus, we then have to be capable of an overt action. The mental aspect of reaction, then, refers to its receptive aspect, the part of us that receives impressions and is capable of, or sensitive to, interpreting or responding to those impressions. When we instinctively react to a loud noise, we have to hear that noise and interpret it; when that happens the reaction has begun. But the pen that has been placed in Richard's hand is not a stimulus unless he makes it one; this reaction should not normally happen and only does so because he has become subconsciously preoccupied with the pen. His reaction to the pen, which is a variation of normal ideo-motor action and not an instinctive reaction, is based on a propensity to become fixated on the pen—to make it into a stimulus because his reaction entails a tendency to become mentally fixated on, or receptive to, the pen as a stimulus.

In order to fully understand the psychology of Richard's problem, then, we have to understand his reaction as a psychological complication of the normal associative process of ideo-motor action. Harmful reaction involves a breakdown of the normal ideo-motor pathway, and its correction requires the readjustment of the physical mechanism as well as the calming down of the system. But to be a reaction, ideo-motor action has to involve not simply an overactive variation of normal ideo-motor action but a complication of the associations which trigger that action. In other words, the reaction is a complication of the normal working of the associative mental process operating to produce motor acts, and this involves a distinctly psychological component.

This psychological complication, to a trained eye, is not difficult to perceive. When Richard looks at the pen, he is guided not by an alert, active interest in the object which is presented to him. He is distracted by the pen; his eyes become lackluster and distant. In short, he is not interested in the pen so much as hypnotized by it. This quality in the eyes is a crucial indicator of what is happening at the mental level and of the importance of this mental level to Richard's overall ability to become aware of and control his actions. Whenever someone is under the influence of a harmful reactive condition, the eyes show a glazed, hypnotic quality, a kind of stupor or lethargy in the level of attention being brought to the task at hand. This distracted, hypnotic quality indicates the presence of psychological preoccupation—a complication of the subconscious process involved in action. If Richard's action had not betrayed his preoccupation with the pen in any other way, his eyes alone would indicate the presence of a harmfully reactive state.

Richard's tendency to react, then, involves a harmful condition not simply of his overall mechanism but of his mental state. In order to be reactive, Richard must be preoccupied in some way, and this indicates the presence of a harmful psychological as well as physical condition. The physical pattern of tension that interferes with the way the body is designed to work is therefore psychologically complex, not simply because it is linked with ideas, but because the mental condition associated with those ideas has become complicated. To fully appreciate the mind/body relationship as it pertains to action, it is critical to understand the psychology of reaction itself.

One can also think of this problem in terms of what a reaction is. Usually we think of a reaction as the act that happens in response to something—a gun goes off, and we are startled by the noise. The reaction, in other words, refers to the startle pattern that is evoked by the noise. But a reaction is a reaction *to something.* The noise has to be interpreted as a noise; otherwise, we would have no reason to react.

In the case of reaction to a loud noise, there is little question about how to interpret this stimulus. This isn't to say that we don't interpret it; in fact, there is a stage of infancy where a child, when presented with an object such as a ball, doesn't know what a ball is and has to learn not just to grab the ball, but to actually interpret its own experience in such a way that it constructs that ball, realizes there is one. But that process is more or less a fixed, developmental sequence; once that sequence has taken place, objects are universally recognized, leaving little room for interpretation.

In the case of voluntary action, however, we have to interpret the pen as something to react to in order for the reaction to take place, and that isn't a fixed process for all people. The person who is calm, relaxed, and alert might not even think to react to that stimulus; if so, he won't become subconsciously fixated on it. When Richard reacted, however, he had to interpret that pen as a stimulus; he had to receive it subconsciously as an impression and become fixated on it, which was the beginning of the reaction itself. That aspect of the reaction—the process of constituting the pen as a stimulus—is the complication of the subconscious idea in the ideo-motor pattern, the mental preoccupation or fixation that takes place at a subconscious level.

When we become subconsciously preoccupied, then, this indicates a distortion of the stimulus, or mental aspect of the stimulus-response pattern. It implies an increased subconscious domination, a propensity to be "caught" by an idea as the beginning of a harmful pattern of reaction. The harmful or reactive working of the ideo-motor pattern indicates that the organism itself is functioning in such a way that it mentally interprets stimuli *as* stimuli. It means not just that we tend to react, but that we interpret situations as stimuli to react to that shouldn't normally attract our attention to begin with.

In practical terms, this means that reaction is significant, not just because of the harmful muscular activity that is associated with it, but because it takes place at all. Remember that Richard isn't simply responding to a stimulus; he is reacting, or responsive, to a stimulus that someone else would not react to to begin with. I tell him I don't want him to stand up out of the chair, and I know that getting out of the chair is precisely what he is going to become fixated on, at a subconscious level. He makes a decision not to speak, but he gets the idea to speak and does so in spite of himself. In short, he continues to interpret situations that in themselves are neutral as if they were a reason to react—in other words, his response pattern means that he is too easily mentally preoccupied or subconsciously captivated by a stimulus.

The harmful pattern of use, then, signifies not only that the ideo-motor pattern is harmfully active and reactive, but that Richard is in a state that makes him respond even when he shouldn't and doesn't want to. It is this fact that explains why Richard is triggered so easily into activity, and why, when we moved him out of a chair, we could produce an action in him by suggesting it. The harmful pattern of activity means literally that Richard is going to get the idea to do things more easily than if the pattern weren't present. In a very practical sense, this means that Richard is going to do more things, and do them more often, than someone who is not reactive. When he speaks, he will tend to follow his own train of associations; while performing tasks at work, he will tend to overreact to situations and to overwork and have trouble stopping when the job is done. His tendency to react in a harmful way means that he reacts more in a purely quantitative sense. A harmfully reactive tendency *in* speaking implies a harmful tendency *to* speak.

This tendency also explains why the normal mechanism of ideo-action we described earlier seemed to be explained by an abnormal pattern of tension. Ideo-motor action, as we saw earlier, is not easy to detect, since most ideas do not issue into action and so are not easily connected with motor acts. Richard's reactive tendency, however—which involved a tendency to be too easily triggered into activity—exposed the link between idea and motor act in a way that made it clearly discernible. Seeing that this ideo-motor mechanism accounted for all voluntary activity, it was then logical to assume that the tension, which was part of this observable mechanism, was therefore part of normal ideo-motor function. We now know that this reaction was not normal ideo-motor action but an example of the harmful working of ideo-motor action. The reaction high-lighted the link between idea and motor act; but once having made that connection, it was necessary to sort out the normal from the abnormal components. The tensions, we now know, don't account for the ideo-motor response; they are part of the reactive pattern that is an exaggeration, or disturbance, of the normal ideo-motor response.

We are now in a position to view the problem of reaction more fully. We initially observed a pattern of tension that interfered with normal postural function. We then saw that this tension was linked with ideas in motor acts, and that this pathway of activity was itself reactive and therefore associated with disturbance. Now that we have compared normal ideo-motor action to reaction, however, we can see that this reactive pattern involves a complication and disturbance in the mental as well as physical elements involved in the basic ideo-motor function, constituting a harmful and uncontrolled tendency in behavior.

Perceiving the mental element in the response reveals yet another aspect of the tendency to separate mind and body. We observed earlier that a simple action such as getting out of a chair or grabbing a pen is viewed in one of two ways. When seen as a muscular action, or as a reaction, it is viewed as bodily. When seen from the point of view of the choice that has been made, the body is seen to be obeying the will or personality of the person "inside" the body. (As we saw, there is no inner "will" governing the act; the muscular response and the mental choice are part of the same process.) When we understand the reaction to include the element of mental receptivity to the stimulus, we can then perceive an even greater intimacy between mind and body. The action is clearly physical, since it involves muscular action and shares some of the characteristics of instinctive reaction. But it is also psychologically complex, since it occurs as the result of a preoccupation with a stimulus that shouldn't normally trigger the action—an intensification of the ideo-motor act. The tension pattern, then, *is* the response itself, the tendency to get the idea and to react intensely. The mind does not affect the body; the response is as much a mental fact as a physical one, because it represents the tendency to become preoccupied with a stimulus that wouldn't even be one if the tension pattern weren't present.

It is also interesting to note that the reaction itself—the tendency to be agitated, to perform the action too quickly, and the emotional state of worry or distraction that is associated with the reaction—would be easily identifiable to the average person. But to the extent that we do notice these reactive qualities, we would, for the most part, designate them as personality traits or expressions of emotions, not as functions in their own right. Once we properly conceive of this type of reaction as a variation of ideo-motor action, however, it becomes clear that these qualities fall not within the domain of psychopathology but within that of the psychology of the unified working of the organism. These traits are not bodily expressions of emotions, but part of the functional psychology of mind and body.

It is not difficult to understand why the view that emotions are expressed in the body is so predominant. I said in the last section that because we typically view stress as a physical expression of emotions, the functioning of the organism is for all intents and purposes ignored. Techniques for controlling tension or reducing stress accordingly borrow psychosomatic concepts to address one end of the spectrum, and relaxation techniques to address the other. Problems are either mental or physical: if the former, we work on emotions; if the latter, the problem is referred to medical treatment or therapy. Putting the two together is then thought to constitute an adequate approach to mind and body.

To be sound, however, a theory of stress must address the organism as a mental and physical whole, and this is why an understanding of reaction is so central to a theory of stress. In order to concretely address Richard's stress, the standard of reaction must itself become the object of study; the physical condition is no longer symptomatic of other factors but is itself the problem. In the context of this problem, emotion represents not the cause of problems, as it does in the field of psychopathology, but very simply must be seen in the context of reaction in living. In short, certain emotional states must be viewed within the context of a unified concept of mind and body.

The unified or psychophysical nature of reaction, then, is an essential component of the problem of stress that we examined in the last section. We observed at that point that agitated or distracted behavior was always thought to be caused by an outside agent or was regarded as symptomatic of deeper psychological causes. The physical state is then thought to be the result of stress—the symptom of a problem which lay elsewhere. We are so accustomed to think that stress and worry are "carried" in our bodies that, in spite of an intellectual acceptance of mind/body unity, we assume that if we have reacted unduly to the stresses at work, such stress is the result of pressures that have caused us to react this way. Accordingly, we deal with stress by reversing the harmful effects we believe it has produced in us.

Disturbance that is associated with reaction, however, cannot be treated except in the context of addressing the reactions of which it is a part. Neurotic behavior may be caused by emotional factors, but the harmful reaction associated with everyday living occurs as part of the functioning of mind and body as a unified whole; no amount of introspection, analysis of causes, or insight into the past can solve a problem that by definition must be addressed in the immediate present, as a matter of actual awareness and control. In this context, emotional elements do not precede or cause tension and reaction, but are associated with the working of the organism as a functional whole.

In concrete terms, the central role of reaction in stress means that the functioning organism, and not emotional "issues," must become the focal point of study in practical attempts to increase awareness and control of mind and body. When we study simple actions such as standing or sitting, it is difficult to imagine that such mundane actions can possibly be significant for our emotional or even physical health; we are more accustomed to attributing problems to emotional or developmental causes. But the organism involved in performing these simple acts is a very complex mental and physical machinery, and the quality of reaction and the associated emotional states are completely dependent on how this organism works in activity. The act of writing *per se* may be mundane, but the complex organism involved in performing this act affects functioning at many levels. In short, the simple, physical acts of standing, walking, and writing—if we understand the basic behavioral functions of which they are a part—is intimately involved in our psychological well-being.

The mechanism of reaction, then, may seem to be of only peripheral interest to psychology. But when we consider the quality of functioning of this mechanism, these mundane actions assume a much greater importance to our general well-being than we would normally attribute to them. If reaction is associated with the way we perform everyday acts, then the quality of functioning in performing these acts is of central interest to our psychological well-being and to the study of psychology generally.

This is an important concept because, until now, emotion has played such a central role in psychology that to say that it is not the primary cause of emotional disturbance almost appears to be a denial of well-established views about the causes of illness and abnormal behavior. In some cases, such a point of view can constitute just such a denial. If, for instance, Susan (returning to our earlier example) demonstrated anxiety or psychosomatic symptoms of stress, one would suspect underlying emotional reasons for her problem. Such is often the case. There are many people whose level of stress and reactivity is so high, and whose emotional distress so plain, that there can be no doubt that the underlying problem is emotional and must be addressed through psychotherapy or other forms of psychiatric treatment.

Such cases, however, do not fall within the domain of the study of mind and body but belong more properly within the field of psychopathology. Where emotion does play a central or primary role, it is the teacher's responsibility to recognize and acknowledge the limitations of knowledge and techniques that will not adequately address such problems. But in the area of normal, everyday stress, emotion is not the primary problem, and working on it directly as the "cause" of the condition of stress will not address the disturbance associated with reaction. In the mind/body area, we must hold to the unified conception where the psychology of reaction, and not emotion, is the central concept.

The same principle holds true for the problem of relaxation. It may be possible, through the practice of methods, to reverse the ill effects of stress, thereby creating the illusion that the problem has been solved. But relaxation—even when it is brought about through a heightened awareness—will not fundamentally alter the pattern of reaction or the stress associated with it, because nothing will have been done to restore the normal working of the ideo-motor pattern with which the stress is associated. The stress that Richard feels, and which he attributes to the difficulties in his work day, are in fact the result of the lack of control and the imbalanced way of doing things that he brings to his activities. When once we understand the psychology of reaction as a unified function, we can no longer attribute symptoms to outside factors but must instead recognize the fundamental educational problem of controlling human reaction as the basis for a true theory of mind and body.

Understanding the psychology of reaction is thus essential to preventing the harmful pattern of tension and gaining an increased awareness and control in activity. If reaction is associated with a complication of the subconscious activity which leads to action, then it is not possible to prevent these reactions simply by becoming kinesthetically aware of the reaction as a pattern of tension. The mental state itself must be addressed by raising the level of alertness and reducing the subconscious preoccupation which leads to uncontrolled reactions.

Addressing the problem of stress is therefore not as simple as it first appears. Clearly, the physical state must be improved by reducing bodily tensions and stress. This is precisely what many stress-reduction methods seek to do by encouraging a reduction in muscular and mental activity. However, these improvements must be accompanied by a heightened awareness which makes it possible not simply to improve the bodily condition, but to become free of the subconscious activity which is at the root of the stressful condition. All too often, stress-reduction techniques have the opposite effect. In the process of reducing stress, the mental state is dulled and awareness reduced. This has the effect not of lowering the subconscious activity associated with stress, but leaving this activity unchecked and even complicating it further. This means that methods that bring about a reduction of stress often perpetuate the causes of the very condition they are attempting to remove by dulling the mind and further deranging the subconscious activity associated with harmful reaction.

It is not sufficient, then, to practice methods which lower stress and improve the bodily condition, however beneficial this may appear. It is necessary to become aware in the present moment by heightening awareness and reducing the subconscious activity associated with mental distraction and preoccupation. We have only to observe the alert intelligence of a young child to understand that mental alertness, and not hypnotic or relaxed states, is the key to relaxation and an absence of stress. An alert, vital awareness is the *sine qua non* of balance in living. Once we conceive the problem in these broader, educational terms, it is clear that hypnosis and other forms of relaxation, by relinquishing the intelligent mind, achieve their results at the expense of the larger educational goal of increased awareness and control in living.

The concept of a balanced mind and body is crucial also to the problem of diagnosis. Since Susan clearly suffered from the effects of stress and nervous agitation, it was difficult to ignore her harmful emotional state. Richard's condition, however, was not nearly so obvious. Although he felt a need to recover from the effects of stress, his actual condition did not appear to be harmful until we viewed it as a pathway of harmful activity. We could then see that rather than being caused by outside factors, his problem was associated with his own harmful functioning. The reactive condition, then, is present in Richard, even when there is no overt symptom, and this is what makes the problem of reaction so central to the study of mind and body. Most mind/body techniques are intended to address the problem of stress by reducing its ill effects, and the belief in therapeutic techniques for reversing the harmful effects of stress is so strong that the need to arrive at a positive concept of health is forgotten entirely. We are so accustomed to addressing problems only when they are serious enough to be regarded as outright clinical symptoms that we fail to see that the real issue is to understand how we are meant to function and how to maintain a balanced state of health. Part of the problem, as we have seen, can be attributed to the fact that many mind/body theories tend to borrow from existing fields, and as such lack their own positive conception of mind and body as a functioning whole. The observation of symptoms is, therefore, bound to be crude: we often wait for outright disaster before we address our state of health. We are bound to be drawn, when presented with a problem to be solved, to precisely those symptoms that are most in need of curing, and we also assume these symptoms—and not a positive understanding of how the organism functions—hold the key to their cure. Consequently, our mind/body systems are based on the study of pathology and are more adept at treating symptoms than at tracing the origins of disturbance.

Once we view reaction as a functional whole, however, we can begin to appreciate the development of these factors in childhood and positively address them based on sound knowledge of how we are designed to function. The beginnings of loss of control, harmful muscular tension, the susceptibility to being triggered into action, the wrong manner of doing things, the reactive mental condition—all these harmful tendencies begin in childhood and can be clearly observed to develop unchecked throughout the life span. To the extent that someone exhibits the pattern of tension and the tendency, which goes hand in hand with it, to manifest the signs of overreaction and disturbance in behavior generally, some degree of breakdown in control, some behavioral disturbance can be said to exist. To a trained observer, such signs are crucial indicators of health; as long as they are ignored, they are bound to develop into outright symptoms, and no therapeutic technique, however effective in addressing such symptoms, will be capable of attacking the root causes of such a problem.

The significance of the concept of reaction, then, is that it provides a positive conception that makes it possible to rise above the need to alleviate symptoms and enables us to aim, instead, at a truly educational approach to well-being. What is needed is an understanding of how we are meant to function and how to maintain not just freedom from illness, but health. A vital physical condition, an alert, positive mental attitude, a balanced level of reaction and calmness in action—all these are qualities that constitute a normal mode of functioning and that serve as a model to guide our efforts to restore normal function. We once ignored mental and emotional factors in health, and yet now have a rich conceptual understanding of the factors that enter into a child's development. We once ignored the role of physical education in the health of the child, and now have at least a concept of what is considered an acceptable standard of fitness. It is now within our power to take into account how the child functions as a mental and physical whole and to insist upon a normal standard of action and reaction as the basis for healthy psychophysical development in the developing child.

The Behavioral Aspect of Reaction

I said in the beginning of this book that many stress-reduction methods promise to eliminate symptoms, but exhibit a lack of clarity about the causes of stress. Many of the inferences that have been drawn about such problems as back trouble have proceeded from subjective perceptions that, as we've seen, presuppose certain biases, such as the idea that back tension, not being directly linked to behavior, emanates from emotional causes. Scientific knowledge, thus far, has been based mainly on empirical studies that, having little regard for the origin of the problem, test the effects of a particular method and base claims of progress on purely therapeutic results.

We have had to do better. Observing how the mind and body function together in action and reaction, we now know that it simply isn't sufficient to make inferences, based on symptoms, about how "mind" affects "body," but to observe, as an actual organism, the working of the muscular system, in what way its functioning has been disturbed, and what elements must come under control in order to restore its normal functioning. By doing this, we have seen how the organism works as a mental and physical whole, how symptoms that appear to us to be caused by other factors are associated with one's own actions and reactions, and how these actions occur subconsciously. In short, a range of symptoms links directly to actions that, having a complex mental and physical basis, must be described in psychological terms if we are to understand their origin.

There is, however, one more aspect of action and reaction that we must observe before we can conclude with a look at the problem of consciousness and conscious control. We've seen that Richard's harmful pattern of activity interfered with the innate working of his muscular system, and that this harmful pattern had to be prevented in order to remove the interference. As he became aware of this pattern, the muscular system and its overactive state began to calm down, revealing the connection of his own actions with a disturbed condition of stress and strain. This makes it possible for Richard, during a series of sessions, to become increasingly quiet and balanced, and to gain increasing control over his actions.

This change, though, is not permanent. If, for instance, Richard is relatively calm one day, when he arrives for the next session he is again worked up or in a state of stress. Even when after a series of sessions the condition of tension is again reduced and the system is finally able to calm down, on subsequent days his system is again in a heightened state of activity, and he has reverted to a reactive and overwrought condition.

At first, it is easy to assume that because the only way to initially help Richard is by making physical adjustments, he simply needs more re-educational work, in order for these problems to be fully eradicated. And in fact, that is to some extent true, since (as we've seen all along) the physical changes are the basis for perceiving—and therefore changing—the harmful pattern of activity. Yet if that were the only requirement, Richard's progress would follow a steady course, and he would slowly arrive at a more desirable condition of relaxed and balanced activity. But that is not the case. If Richard has been on vacation, he is in a markedly calm state, whereas if he has spent an entire day at the computer, or meeting a pressured schedule at work, he is noticeably tense and worked up. In other words, his condition fluctuates depending on what he has been doing.

It soon becomes clear that Richard's state of tension, and the activities he has been engaged in, are very closely related. If he has just finished a project at work, he is somewhat overwrought. If, in contrast, he has just come back from vacation, his condition is noticeably calmer. He may realize, in the former case, that he is uncomfortable and overwrought, but, because he has been too busy to notice how he became tense, he experiences his problem as physical and is therefore unlikely to perceive the role he has himself played in causing his problem. After a number of sessions, however, it becomes clear that his condition is directly related to what he has been doing, and that this factor is crucial to gaining control over the problem.

This daily context represents a new layer of the problem that we haven't yet explicitly dealt with. We've seen so far that the pattern of muscular tension is related to action, making it necessary to look at the psychology of how action takes place. Next, we saw that the overall working of the system was interfered with, causing Richard to react in a way that was harmful. These observations involved us in a detailed examination of how ideas and muscular tension are involved to produce action, and how this system becomes complicated or disturbed.

But to say that the ideo-motor system is working wrong is to make a statement about behavior itself, since the function of ideo-motor action is to produce behavior. If, for instance, Richard's back has become harmfully tense, it is tempting to think that the pattern of ideo-motor action explains why the back tightens during the day. However, it would be just as accurate to say that since ideo-motor action *is* behavior, the recurring act of tightening his back causes a disturbance in the ideo-motor pattern.

The same is true with the problem of reaction. Richard's tendency to jump out of the chair in an uncontrolled manner was caused by a harmful condition of the functioning of his ideo-motor mechanism, which, as we saw, was related to a breakdown in the inhibitory aspect of activity. But if Richard tends to be reactive in jumping out of the chair, then he will also tend to be reactive in daily living, which is the true context of these reactions. When viewed in this way, neither factor can be said to cause the other. If the mechanism that governs behavior is imbalanced, then behavior itself will be imbalanced.

Richard's symptoms, then, represent a problem not simply in how his behavioral mechanism works, but in his actual behavior. Richard assumes his "condition" can be therapeutically corrected—that is, rectified by seeking professional help by an expert. But he spends hours every day in a more or less uncontrolled state, and has done so for years, and this means that his condition, or the way he is functioning, is directly connected with his own activity. In fact, in each case I've described, the wrong functioning of the mechanism always manifests, to some degree, in a condition of stress that is associated with an uncontrolled way of living, of conducting oneself, in daily life. We are all familiar with not being able to stop at the end of the day. We think about the day's events; thoughts turn over in our brain; we grind our jaw; we cannot unwind. This is what is happening in Richard after he has engaged in a typical day's work. His disturbed condition indicates that he has become worked up and can't stop, and it manifests, at the end of the day, in a disturbed condition that, in this sense, is merely symptomatic of the larger problem of behavior itself.

This explains the real root of Richard's problem. When he is in a disturbed condition, he is not aware of his own harmful actions, his rushing, his preoccupied mental state. He only knows at the end of the day that he needs to unwind, that he must get away from the environment that "causes" this tension. But the stress Richard experiences is caused by his own reactions to this environment—reactions that take the form of increasingly uncontrolled behavior during these periods of increased pressure. Although work seems to "cause" the stress, it is Richard's own actions and reactions that are the problem.

This behavioral component represents a critical aspect of the problem of the control of reaction. Earlier, we observed that the ideo-motor mechanism is designed to work in a fluid and unconscious manner, so that it is possible to get things done, to perform actions, without having to think about *how* we perform each and every action. This makes it inherently difficult, even for someone who is attempting to be aware of this system, to perceive what he is doing. Being aware of one's actions is even more difficult when, as in Richard's case, action is rushed, uncontrolled, and reactive. By looking at this mechanism in the context of Richard's daily lifestyle, we can now see the full implications of what is meant by unified activity of mind and body. When we consider that ideo-motor action is the mechanism by means of which we perform the actions of daily life, then an overactive ideo-motor pathway implies imbalanced activity in daily life. Imbalanced conduct is itself the cause of Richard's overwrought condition.

Gaining awareness and control of this behavioral dimension of reaction is critical to understanding the mental and emotional attitudes at the root of stress. To the extent that certain situations create emotional stress, it is fair to say that in order to reduce the stress a change in attitude and emotion is required. But the stress associated with reaction cannot be removed by exploring emotions directly. If, for instance, Richard became aware of the emotional attitude connected with his reaction to deadlines at work, the reaction itself would not cease: he would still become overwrought after a day's work, and his actions would still tend to be uncontrolled. Perhaps most important, he would not be able to change the deterioration in mental and emotional attitude that happens, as we saw a moment ago, as a result of becoming overwrought. Because we think of reaction as a response to a particular stimulus, it is easy to assume that the stress is the physical response to an emotional stimulus, the bodily condition therefore being the result of some outside "cause." But stress is associated with reaction, not caused by it; and the only way to control our own harmful reactions is to gain control of behavior itself.

Richard thinks, then, that if he relaxes, or changes his emotional attitude, he can reverse his stressful condition. But his own unconscious and uncontrolled behavior and misdirected way of doing things over time have led to his condition of stress. Stress doesn't simply "happen," and it isn't caused by something "out there." When Richard is engaged in the bustle of daily life—paying his bills, driving to work—he is reacting to something, but the reaction isn't a physical reaction to an emotional attitude. When properly understood, reaction is itself the problem, and since reaction occurs in daily life, it is necessary to understand his own action and how it operates as the basis for achieving psychophysical balance.

Understanding—and taking responsibility for—the actual behavioral patterns with which emotional attitudes are associated represents the basis of a true psychology of stress, and its true application is in the field not of therapy but of education. It is necessary, as part of the process of gaining control of behavior, to alter one's attitudes and beliefs. But these attitudes and beliefs are associated with reaction itself and cannot be fully understood through introspection alone. In this context, conceiving the mind/body connection as the influence of emotions over the body, and of a psychology based on this interactionist concept, is inadequate to address the problem of stress. It is necessary, instead, to frame a new psychology of mind and body as a subconsciously functioning whole that must be brought under conscious control.

Understanding this behavioral dimension of reaction also clarifies what we mean when we speak of tension caused by everyday stresses. We commonly assume that when we become tense the tension is a "buildup" from the day's activities, that emotions manifest in the body, and that we consequently "carry" or "hold" tensions that are brought about by emotional stress. But everyday tension is in fact symptomatic of a problem not with the body or emotions but with our own behavior, and that is why methods designed to release tension are not adequate to address the problem.

Part of the difficulty in perceiving the relationship between tension and behavior again harks back to the separation we make between mind and body. Take, as an illustration, the case of a driver who pulls the head back and strains the neck and shoulders while driving. Earlier, we saw that, in performing a physical movement, tension is part of a total mental and physical process. Because driving is a relatively inert activity, it is easy to assume that the driver's tension, like a startle pattern, is a physical reaction to the stress of driving. Close observation reveals, however, not only that the driver is tense, but that he is rushing, preoccupied, and overinvolved, and this is the clue to what is really happening. Driving is, first and foremost, a voluntary act requiring a complex process of perception, association, and physical response, and muscular activity is part of that total process. The tensed attitude of the driver may seem to be a reaction *to something,* but the tension is in fact part of the driver's own misdirected tendency to behave, in this case, in an uncontrolled way. The tension, then, isn't just a reactive physical response that vaguely relates to being wound up, so that the mind or emotional factors mysteriously "express" themselves, or are "held," in the driver's tensed body. The tension pattern is in fact the observable side of the total activity of driving occurring in an uncontrolled, overstimulated way.

When we speak of tensing "in response to a situation," or a situation "making us tense," this often represents a misunderstanding of what is actually happening. Tension is an indication that the physical mechanism is working wrong; in this sense, there is a purely physical aspect of the problem. But tension occurs as part of voluntary activity, not as a by-product of it. It might be accurate to speak of tension as a reaction when we experience trauma or become startled. But in everyday activities such as driving, tension is part of the total pathway of muscular and physical activity.

Making this connection between tension and behavior is critical to properly addressing the cause of tension. We saw, in the earlier chapter on ideo-motor action, that tension is in fact part of a total mental and physical process of activity. But it is in the context of real life, when the activity becomes uncontrolled and overactive, that the tension occurs in its worst form. When we speak of tension as an expression of something else, we are ignoring the central role of our own behavior, and end up treating the tension separately in the form of relaxation and winding-down exercises. As a result, we misdiagnose the problem, not simply because we don't see tension as part of a total mental and physical process, but because we don't see it as part of behavior. Nothing is causing the driver to tense up; the tension is the result of his own behavior. The driver's problem cannot be addressed adequately by methods that treat a "condition." The only solution is to raise this entire activity to a conscious level, by adopting a conscious attitude toward living.

Notice also that "behavior" isn't always an overtly physical activity. Driving may be relatively sedentary, but it is nevertheless a total activity; like speaking, walking, or cooking, it involves a complex process of thinking, perceiving, responding, and physically moving. If the driver tenses in response to getting at the wheel, the tension is an indication not so much of some outside "stress" that causes that tension but of loss of control, of rushing, of preoccupation—even when that rushing and loss of control do not manifest in overt actions such as walking or typing quickly. The same can be said of reading, solving problems, or working at a computer. In these activities the mental functions predominate, and so it is particularly easy to separate the physical element of stress from the activity itself. But just observe a computer user as he becomes involved in working at a computer, and the real problem becomes apparent: his eyes glaze over, he "loses" himself in what he is doing, and he no longer takes time but becomes almost obsessive in getting things done. Here, the involvement is largely mental and, as with many intellectual occupations, the uncontrolled reactions exhibit themselves mainly in the form of an unhealthy degree of overinvolvement in, or preoccupation with, the task at hand. But working at a computer is nevertheless a total activity in which a stimulus, or the idea to do something, has led to a series of associations and responses—in other words, a total mental and physical activity—and it is this entire pathway of action that must come under control.

Seeing the problem of ideo-motor action and its wrong reactive working in our everyday actions begins to place the problem of reaction in the context of actual living. In an earlier section I said that all of Richard's actions—or at least all of his voluntary actions—can be accounted for on the basis of the ideo-motor pattern, in which an idea triggers a motor act. We then saw that this activity involved increasing disturbance in the functioning of this mechanism, involving a complication of the subconscious mental process and harmful or uncontrolled reactions. We have now established the behavioral context of this process and its operation in day-to-day living. The standard of functioning of the mechanism means a particular condition that can be observed in a clinical context, but it also implies a mode of conduct, of day-to-day behavior.

This behavioral dimension, however, is not immediately apparent, even to the skilled observer. If Richard sees a professional for help, the professional must view him in an artificial situation, where by definition Richard is removed from the stresses of work and therefore does not exhibit the agitation or rushing associated with his professional life. Clinically speaking, however, it is the teacher's job to observe Richard's actions and, in so doing, to infer what reactions in everyday life may be contributing to his condition. By perceiving a loss of control in, say, raising an arm or in speech, a clear picture begins to emerge, revealing a link between Richard's condition and what he is actually doing in daily life. Whenever there is a breakdown in the ability to stop, however mundane the activity in which this tendency manifests; whenever there is an overexcitability in speech, or a tendency to become mentally preoccupied while forming thoughts or while performing some simple action—

in each of these cases there will be a corresponding loss of control or imbalance in daily living that will, to a greater or lesser degree, manifest as a stressful condition in living.

The most obvious indicator of the connection between stress and behavior is the hustle and bustle of street life. It is not difficult, simply observing people walking down a city street, to note how many people habitually rush through the day's activities, anxiety and worry written on their faces. This is the most obvious sign of imbalance, but it isn't difficult to observe mental preoccupation, impatience, the compulsion to get something done, and the general state of nervous exhaustion that is so universal in city-dwellers. It is also fairly easy to observe how much effort some people require to perform simple tasks, and the tendency, once having finished the job, to collapse—evidence of a lack of moderation that so often leads to a debilitated mental and physical condition. The same lack of moderation can be observed in people who live between the extremes of over-working and exercising strenuously and then collapsing or practicing a form of relaxation in the attempt to recover from the state of tension in which they find themselves.

Insomnia, mentioned in the section on reaction and stress, is another form of disturbance directly connected with behavior. If behavior is uncontrolled during waking hours, it is little wonder that, when we intend to stop at the end of the day, we find we cannot. In this sense insomnia reflects immoderation not during sleep but during the day's activities: the disturbance associated with the activity persists even when the organism is not engaged in overt activity.

These forms of loss of control are just a few of the qualities that can be observed in modern life. Needless to say, there are many other factors, such as emotional illness, overwork, and financial pressures, that contribute to stress and disturbance. In many cases, it requires a good deal of experience to distinguish harmful forms of reaction from pathological conditions associated with emotional disorders; often a number of factors are at work. The practical reality of addressing harmful states of stress, however, demands not simply treatment of the condition but attention to conduct itself. It is the teacher's job to understand this connection between stress and conduct and, in so doing, to encourage the student to take responsibility not just for how he performs actions but for his entire lifestyle.

We have now uncovered the problem of "use" in its many layers. We initially observed action as a physical pattern of tension that interfered with the body's natural system of support and balance. We then connected this pattern of tension to a mental and physical pathway of activity in which action is produced. We then examined this pattern in the context of harmful reaction and emotional states. All of these steps related to a clinical situation independent of daily life and could be reduced to a single observable movement or set of movements. When we relate this activity to its true context in daily behavior, however, we can see clearly how the entire problem demands not therapy or treatment but knowledge and conscious awareness of conduct. Mind/body methods, properly applied, belong not in the field of medicine or therapy but in the domain of education.

The behavioral aspect of ideo-motor action also provides another level of explanation of how the problem develops. A moment ago, I said that when Richard is overwrought or in a condition of stress, it isn't always to the same degree. When he has just come back from a vacation, he is relatively calm and focused. Within a week or so of returning to work, however, he is again overwrought and again exhibits a loss of control in actions that he performs repeatedly at work. This connection with behavior, we saw, indicated that reaction can't be separated from behavior: they are two ways of speaking about the same thing.

But why does the reaction develop at work to begin with? At first, the answer seems to be simply that work itself is stressful and therefore causes Richard to react to this stress by becoming tense; that would explain the difference between Richard's condition at work and on vacation. But there are two factors which militate against this explanation. First, returning from vacation does not in itself cause the level of reaction we have observed. It is only after he has been at work for a period of time, and becomes preoccupied and rushed, that the reaction level actually increases.

Second, and perhaps more important, a demanding and pressured job does not, in itself, cause the kind of problem we have been speaking about. It is only after someone has been engaged in a particular occupation for a period of years that the level of reaction usually becomes harmful. We have only to observe how people deteriorate with age to confirm this. If, for instance, you observe a pianist at the beginning of his career, his level of reaction—even when he plays with too much tension—will be relatively low. After he has performed year in and year out in the same way, though, his actions become increasingly uncontrolled, and his overall condition deteriorates to the point where he becomes quite literally disturbed.

These facts suggest that another factor is at work. The condition that is associated with Richard's harmful way of doing things is disturbed, but it is the actual fact of doing things over time—his tendency to rush at work, to respond too quickly when engaged in conversation, to talk on the phone in a hurried manner, to hurry through the details of each workday—that brings about the harmful condition. Reaction and behavior are quite inseparable, but the breakdown in reaction cannot itself occur except over time, through a process of deterioration. In other words, it is Richard's own behavior, his own way of responding to the stress of work, that causes the disturbance to intensify over time.

This adds a new dimension to our understanding of the development of the problem. Earlier, I spoke about how, as a child, the functional stability of the ideo-motor response breaks down until, with time, actions become more and more reactive and uncontrolled. But if it is correct to say that the inhibitory function breaks down, it is equally correct to say that behavior itself breaks it down: it is the fact of doing things, day in and day out, that actually causes the mechanism to get more and more imbalanced. Over a period of years, the deterioration increases so that by adulthood, the average person is in a generally disturbed condition and often relies on artificial stimulants and sensory indulgences in order to relax. This statement can be applied to many people, but each person's tendencies follow the course peculiar to his or her individual makeup and circumstances. There is that rare person who stays calm and balanced throughout life, but this fortunate individual belongs to a dying breed, and for the vast majority today, disturbance and nervous strain are the overwhelming fact of everyday life.

This connection between stress and conduct reveals a fundamental aspect of the psychology of action and reaction. In psychology when we speak of a disturbance or pathology, the abnormality is usually located in the individual and is normally thought to inhibit behavior, limit it, put constraints on it, or otherwise distort it; behavior is seen to be the symptom, not the cause. But because reaction occurs in daily life as behavior, then the actual fact of behavior—doing things year after year—itself tends to increase the level of distortion and misdirection. In other words, we normally speak in psychology of pathology affecting behavior; but in the psychology of mind and body, behavior affects functioning. The cause of the problem is literally behavior itself.

This role of behavior in causing the deterioration in the machinery of action brings a new aspect of functioning into focus. In the last section I spoke about how, in contrast to other areas of psychology, the study of use and action constitutes a distinct area of study in which the unified working of the whole holds the key to understanding disturbance associated with reaction. We can now add another factor to this field of study. Since the wrong working of this mechanism manifests in daily living as uncontrolled behavior, then the psychology of action revolves not around the study of pathological conditions but around conduct itself. Normally we don't think of how we live, how we conduct ourselves, as having significance, at least not to our mental or emotional health. Illness manifests itself in our behavior and sometimes forces us to alter our behavior in order to control the illness—the illness being something other than behavior. But because stress is associated with the working of the mechanism of action, our stress level therefore depends upon our own actions and conduct. In this sense, behavior itself, not internal or external causes, must become the focal point in the study of stress.

In order to give this area of functioning its complete due, however, we must fully appreciate its place in human psychology. I said earlier that our attitudes about mind and body reflect a cultural prejudice that values the intellectual over the physical, and that we tend to separate personality from movement and reaction and other tangible bodily functions. This same bias expresses itself in our attitude towards the occupations we value. Along the mind/body spectrum, long-term goals and intellectual activities are valued highly because they correspond to "mind," while immediate enjoyments and simple activities, which correspond to the "body," rate lower on the scale. This attitude is reflected in the low status accorded such behavior in the realm of psychological, emotional, or spiritual health: a child may have the time to indulge in mundane activities, but in the world of adult responsibilities such time is not available and if it is, must be relegated to "higher" pursuits. Understanding conduct in a practical way, however, holds the key to living a balanced existence, free of constant worry and nervous strain. The problem of conduct, far from being trivial or incidental to higher functions, is in fact central to the entire question of stress and strain in living. Nothing is so critical to understanding the problem of everyday stress as the simple fact of our own conduct.

Such an approach also requires a shift in our attitude about illness. A number of mind/body theories have been advanced based on empirical studies that demonstrate a link between mental states and physical symptoms. According to these theories, stress is conceived as a response to objective factors, without reference to the self; and the symptom, which is purely physical, has no reference to the outside world. The stimulus, in other words, is external; our emotional response to it causes the physiological condition of stress.

By observing Richard's behavior as an actual, operational mechanism, and by tracing this behavioral function from our original study of his movement, we have introduced—or perhaps recovered—the self as the essential intermediary factor. The overwrought condition associated with the reactive working of this mechanism, and the nervous strain that we attribute to emotional or external stressors, are in fact one and the same. This makes it possible to understand stress, not as a specific bodily response to an internal or external cause but as part of an overall unhealthy, unconscious condition of response—emotional state included—which requires a conscious attitude toward living.

The study of conduct and its role in illness and functioning represents a vast and, as yet, unrecognized area in psychology. To an untrained observer, bodily action is hardly worthy of study; only students of dance, acting, or martial arts have any reason to give it their attention. To one who understands the functional unity of mind and body, however, awareness of action holds the key to living calmly and deliberately. If you would understand how mind and body work as a psychophysical whole, you must understand the significance of this function to day-to-day living; and if you would understand how to live in a balanced, healthy way, you must understand how the mind and body cooperate in action. The unity of mind and body is significant, not simply because it holds the key to living without physical and nervous strain, but because it provides the basis for living in a conscious and balanced way.

CHAPTER SIX
· · · · · · · ·

Conscious Prevention and Control

The Field of Consciousness

In virtually all the mind/body methods that treat tension and stress, it is possible, through a purely clinical process, to isolate and solve problems without reference to a raising of consciousness of the subject. Even where, as in the practice of meditation or relaxation methods, there is a heightening of consciousness, the process can still be described and practiced clinically, and often does not require self-responsibility at any level other than the practice of the method. But the problem of mind and body as we've seen it is not a pathology, but emanates from our own activity. As such, it cannot be addressed in the mechanistic ways common to medical treatment but must instead take into account one's own behavior. Even an appreciation of the interconnectedness of mind and body is not itself sufficient to address the study of action, which requires a concept of the unified working of mind and body in the context of daily life. The problem of tension and stress, then, cannot ultimately be solved, or described, through clinical practice or any particular kind of treatment; the problem is essentially that of the control of one's own behavior, of how to raise the subconscious process of action to a conscious level.

We have now reached the final stages of the problem. I said, in the beginning, that mind and body are often conceived as two interacting systems, and that by utilizing the connection between these systems, we can improve our health and well-being. In the present context, however, mind and body can be fully understood only in the context of action—as a subconscious activity that must, through an educational process, be brought to consciousness. Ultimately, this problem requires not simply bodily awareness but heightened consciousness in living—a subject I would now like to turn to.

In the last chapter, I said that when Richard initiates an action, his actions are mentally and physical imbalanced. The tension pattern, we then saw, is not only part of an immediate pathway of idea and motor act, but is also connected with an overactive condition associated with stress and disturbance, and complicated by mental preoccupation at a sub-conscious level that makes Richard unable to think and act calmly. It was necessary, in order to address this problem, for Richard to learn to prevent his habitual actions, to act more calmly, and to raise his level of mental awareness. This not only restored his system to a quieter condition but also helped him to recognize the underlying mental preoccupation associated with activity.

But how do these changes relate to consciousness? Let's look once more at the psychology of ideo-motor action. We've seen that muscle action is part of a pathway of activity issuing from ideas; this is their normal function. Which pathway is initiated, we also saw, emerges out of a complex of competing ideas: when one idea weakens, or one grows strong, then the deadlock between competing ideas is broken and action takes place. This shows how ideo-motor action actually occurs. Ideas are always competing for discharge within a complex mental field—the field of consciousness[*]—and action is the result of how this competition is resolved.

The complexity of associations underlying voluntary action explains why it is so difficult to prevent the habitual ideo-motor response from occurring in a complex activity such as typing. The undesirable muscle activity, whether we like it or not, is continually being triggered by the idea of doing something. Under the guidance of a teacher, it is possible to perceive what is happening, because it is a reaction that shouldn't be happening. But because voluntary action invokes the very associative pro-cess that initiates action—and at a level that is largely subconscious—it is virtually impossible to prevent the ideo-motor response from occurring, once one is involved in an activity.

Richard's process of stopping in relation to the impulse to act, how-ever, brings about a quieting of this mental field of activity, and this is a crucial step in raising the normally subconscious process of ideo-motor

[*] Although the word "consciousness" is usually used to denote awareness, in the context of the term "field of consciousness" it refers to something entirely different—namely, the array of ideas that compete for discharge into action.

action to a conscious level. The act of trying not to think about typing, as we saw, still involves thinking about it. This thought process, in turn, was connected with various muscular actions that occurred unconsciously. The process of stopping and noticing these trains of thought, however, leads to a mental quieting and a weakening of the compulsion to act. This, in turn, leads to a quieting of both muscular activity and the mental associations that are subliminally connected with it.

This quieting of mental activity is a crucial element in the process of gaining conscious control over action and reaction. Until now I've spoken about the connection of ideas and motor acts in behavior. I also said that in practice various ideas compete for discharge, comprising a field of consciousness in which one idea will prevail among the various possibilities occurring mentally. (The attempt to type or not to type, as well as the myriad choices occurring during the process of working at a computer, are good examples.) This mental activity, as we've seen, is quite complex, involving mental preoccupation, tension, and overactivity in the system. But all this activity occurs subconsciously, and this explains why, when we try to become aware of the ideo-motor process, we cannot; the field of ideas operates constantly to produce activity at a level of which we are unaware.

When we meet the challenge of preventing the habitual muscular activity, however, this slows down the normal process of doing and the impulse to do, and the mental activity associated with this motor activity quiets down as well. This quieting of mental associative activity—and of the motor activity that goes with it—implies a heightening of conscious awareness. We are not, for the most part, aware of the mental associations taking place; the unconscious worry, concern, and waste of energy is largely subconscious. But when the system becomes quiet, the activity in the field of mental associations subsides, and there is a spontaneous realization that one's mental awareness had been clouded by unnecessary thinking and worrying. Just as a noise to which one has become accustomed goes unnoticed until the moment that it stops, so the "noise" in the mental field is not perceived until the moment that the mind becomes quiet. In its place is a perceptual alertness, a heightened awareness of one's surrounding, and, with the quieting of preoccupying thoughts, a heightened consciousness.

This awareness represents a crucial element in solving the ideo-motor problem. The pattern of ideo-motor activity, we saw earlier, is connected with a harmful pattern of muscular tension. This tension, in turn, implies a state of reaction that must calm down; we saw this happen when the teacher brought about a reduction in this overactivity. But the true context of ideo-motor action is that of voluntary behavior, and this involves mental associations that are in fact part of one's own process of engaging in voluntary activity. Only by becoming conscious in oneself of this activity, and therefore bringing about a quieting of this associative activity, is it possible to alter this process.

This connection of motor activity with the complex associations involved in voluntary action is critical to understanding the role of consciousness in addressing the problem of tension and stress. Methods that utilize consciousness often appeal to the power of consciousness to effect changes in health. These observed changes are then used to support a concept of mind/body unity based on the observed connection between empirical effects and physical improvements. But since disturbance and stress are associated with the organism as an active, responding organism, methods that do not address the need for consciousness as it applies to increased control of the organism in action are failing to address the problem in its true context. Relaxation methods may bring about an increased sense of relaxation or effect other therapeutic changes, but to address the cause of the problem, it is necessary to become increasingly alert and calm, in the context of the associative process that takes place during voluntary action. In short, the subconscious associative process of ideo-motor action must be raised to a conscious level by quieting the field of consciousness.

The true significance of the role of consciousness as it applies to stress in living, then, is not in the context of therapeutic techniques, but as a heightened awareness in living—a conscious stage of functioning. All along, I have insisted on the need not for methods that treat symptoms but for a clear articulation of subject matter that clarifies what causes the problem. As with all the elements we have observed in this book, consciousness must be seen not simply as a therapeutic tool but in the context of its role in human behavior. When the system is disturbed, the normally subconscious process of action must be raised to a conscious level. Obvious as these observations may sound, however, methods which utilize the power of awareness or consciousness to effect physical changes rarely bring about a truly heightened state of consciousness; in fact, they often have the opposite effect. By encouraging a relaxed condition and a "calm" mental state, the underlying mental process, instead of being brought to awareness, is actually left untouched and, in some cases, is actually complicated by an increased tendency to become preoccupied, hypnotically distracted, or otherwise mentally dulled. In order to truly address the problem of consciousness, the underlying mental associations associated with harmful activity must be quieted down in order to bring about a heightened and vital condition of mental alertness.

But why should the field of mental activity quiet down, if the associative process is necessary to ideo-motor action—if, in other words, mental activity is *meant* to take place? Let us look first at the normal role of associations as they take place within the field of consciousness. We saw earlier that ideas are always competing for discharge within a complex field of consciousness, and that action is the result of how this competition is resolved. The complexity of the mental field is further complicated by the fact that ideas do not exist singly but are connected in complex trains of associations. When, earlier, we observed a triggered ideo-motor action, it was specific to an immediate task or movement: getting out of a chair, taking a breath, speaking a phrase, and so on. In real life, however, it is not so simple. When, for instance, we think of getting out of bed in the morning, it is not the movement of getting out of bed *per se* that is confronting us, but rather a more distant and complex set of concerns that require getting out of bed as the first step. This is true in virtually all the acts of daily life. We sit down not because we decide to lower our weight onto a chair, but because we want to read, or rest; we take a breath (in the case of speaking) not because we are conscious of needing to breathe or even because we need air to speak, but because we are conversing on a particular subject and want to express an opinion. The stimuli to act, then, rarely demand specific movements such as we saw earlier in the case of jumping out of the chair, and are aimed instead at more "distant" objectives. Of course, if we get out of bed because we want to take a shower, it is still accurate to say that we intended to get out of bed. The point is that the immediate action is in fact performed in the service of a more distant end.

Ideo-motor action, then, is complicated not simply by the array of ideas that compete for discharge but by the constellation of associations that lead, in any particular case, to a completed act. In each action, we do not intend to perform particular movements; it would be more accurate to say that the need to achieve a distant end brings into play whatever movements are necessary to achieve that end, without thinking about it. Most of the stimuli to act in daily life are in this sense distant: they do not stimulate us to perform particular movements; rather, in order to accomplish the end, we must perform a series of movements involving a complex train of associations. When this occurs, one is not aware of having done the intermediate steps: the specific movements are unthinkingly performed in the service of the larger overall task.

Thus, the associations that occur, even in simple actions, are a complex series of ideas and habits, each linked to the next, and the physical actions necessary to accomplish a particular end are entirely subordinated to this end and performed automatically. From a practical point of view this is important, since when we try to gain control over this process, it is more difficult to prevent the subconscious act of expressing an opinion (the distant end) than to prevent the taking of a breath (immediate end). From a theoretical point of view, it means that the psychological complexity of ideo-motor action is not limited simply to the array of ideas, or choices, that can issue into action, but itself connects up with entire cognitive structures within which action takes place. These cognitive structures are, quite literally, part of the mental world we live in, and it is a complex world indeed.

This connection between complex thinking and action demonstrates the inextricable link between thought process and motor function. It is easy to assume that since ideas do not always issue in action, and since thinking occurs as a distinct human activity, thought processes aren't connected with action. But the capacity to think evolved in the context of action; mental operations or ideas are developments, refinements in the capacity to act and in action itself—not something separate from it. When we think, ideas seem to take on a life of their own; we are capable of thinking as a distinct activity. But ideas are functionally related to action, to motor activity.

This relationship is somewhat clearer when we compare the adult to the child. In a young infant, motor activity is directly linked with thought: an infant is always moving and, within a few months of age, is distracted very easily by any strong stimulus, to which it immediately responds. This is why it is easier to distract an infant than to actually stop its action: its actions occur impulsively in relation to whatever stimuli are present. This constant activity can't be stopped, but it can be redirected by new associations. Later, the child develops increasingly complex cognitive abilities and learns to inhibit its action. But we have to remember that the intelligent and deliberate action of the older child is still a variation, or a refinement, of the original connection between association and motor action. In other words, there is still a link of thought to motor activity, except that the link is obscured by the complexity of mental activity, which creates greater variability of choice.

This relation of thought to motor activity is often overlooked in the study of intelligence and cognition. Typically when we observe human cognitive processes, we forget to look in the active present. We view mind as a "thing," an instrument of thought, and forget that it is a functional process related to behavior. Mental operations have everything to do with living itself; they are not merely a "domain" of subjective meanings and experiences. Seen in this way, we can discern a connection between the muscular system on the one hand—and the way in which it is functioning—and the mental choices and directions our actions take on the other. The so-called body is the physical machinery of this ideo-motor process.

Also, the traditional and much-criticized view of learning—that the mind is a blank slate for accumulating facts—has completely misread how the mind works. We learn things, facts, mainly as a means for action; education that makes facts an end in themselves is not only boring but irrelevant and impractical as well. Nor are most of the things that we know merely facts—that is an illusion, even in people who pride themselves on the vast numbers of facts they have accumulated. Most of the facts that we have committed to memory—knowing where things are, the vast numbers of words in our vocabulary and our facility with language, the ability to discriminate among voices and faces, and so on—are in reality part of learned actions in the context of our daily lives. We don't know that we know most of these things, but they constitute a vast repertoire of knowledge, and they are all related to action. The ability to learn facts, then, is an impressive ability, a kind of virtuoso talent that we claim as a special educational ability or goal. But knowledge, the ability to learn facts, evolved primarily in order to serve action. Mental knowledge is functionally related to action.

The cognitive and associative operations that connect with voluntary action are thus highly complex, and this complexity is inherited as an instinctive function. This explains why it is so difficult, in voluntary action, to change what we are doing, and why the associative process underlying action is so complicated. From an evolutionary point of view, we have inherited the associative process as the basis for action itself, and this complex field is operating habitually as a normal rule, even when we are trying to control or change our actions, or are making deliberate choices.

As we've observed all along, however, this complex field of ideas is not, for the most part, conscious. When, for instance, we get up in the morning, we do not consciously deliberate about which actions to make or notice exactly how we physically rise out of bed or put on our clothes. During the relatively infrequent moments that we think about our actions, we can make a self-fulfilling argument that we are, in fact, conscious of how we do things. But if we are conscious of our actions it is because when we observe what we are doing, we are by definition conscious. In fact, the vast majority of our actions are stereotyped and automatic, and the complex associative processes involved in performing them occur at an almost completely subconscious level.

Part of the reason that our actions are so automatic is because we learn to make them so. As we master particular actions, they become habitual; it is far easier to perform the innumerable actions of daily life routinely than to think about each one. But actions—even apart from the fact that they tend to become habitual with time—are subconscious simply because that is their nature. We are so naturally biased in the direction of assuming consciousness—the things we are aware of—that we have come to believe that unconscious behavior is associated with pathology, denial, or some alteration of consciousness. But such is of course not the case. Action is naturally habitual, naturally unconscious; consciousness is a later development.

This becomes clearer if you consider this problem from an evolutionary perspective. In primitive species action is neither conscious nor unconscious; it just happens, instinctively, automatically. The ability to respond in different ways to the environment implies a more highly developed nervous system, which is what we mean—or certainly one of the things we mean—by mind. At this point, we can speak of having ideas; but action is still habitual, merely less so than when it is completely instinctive. But the fact that an animal can make one action as opposed to another—or its ability to distinguish between alternatives or to make choices—does not mean that its action is willed in the sense that it is consciously determined. Complex actions are no less determined than purely instinctive responses; they simply involve a level of mental processing that is far more cognitively complex than that of purely instinctive actions.

It is therefore a very serious mistake to equate mind with consciousness. Mind is what we mean when we have complex ways of responding to things, or when we perform complex mental operations, but such actions are still as a rule subconscious. Even when—as in the case of humans or other "higher" animals—we are capable of intelligent action, we function at an essentially subconscious level. A brilliant mathematician may be nonetheless unaware of his surroundings, of how he walks or of how to perform even simple motor skills; a seemingly dull intellect may in contrast be calm, deliberate, and possess excellent judgment in general matters of living. In other words, the cognitive elements that we sometimes equate with consciousness presume the subconscious operation of habit; they do not supersede it. This is true, also, of the capacity to make choices. The ability of an animal to choose the maze that will lead to food, or of a human to choose the right answer to a question, presupposes some element of consciousness, but we don't generally make such choices consciously. Animals are capable of making extraordinarily complex decisions when attacking prey, or while searching for food, but these choices are nonetheless made subconsciously. As with animals, most human choices, as well as the reasons for making them, are made subconsciously.

Subconsciousness, then, is an unfortunate word, since it implies something that exists only in relation to consciousness—namely, below it—when it is in fact the rule. Our language reflects our own natural bias. From the point of view of what we actually experience, what is subconscious *is* below consciousness, and to this extent it accurately reflects, if not our actual, at least our subjective experience. By "subconscious," however, I do not mean something subordinate to consciousness. Rather, I mean automatic, ingrained, or implying action that occurs at an instinctive, innate level, and which is therefore not conscious. Such action is the overwhelmingly predominant force in animal and human behavior.

The subconscious associative process, then, is certainly not abnormal; it is *meant* to occur. Without making constant associations, we would not be capable of flexible action; it is precisely this associative complexity that makes us capable of intelligent choice. But in humans, this process becomes psychologically complicated in a way that is *not* normal. Compare, for instance, how ideo-motor action occurs in humans as opposed to animals. Ideo-motor action, as we've seen, is a complex process of choosing from among competing alternatives. The same can be said of animals. When, for instance, a dog walks down the street, there is an overwhelming complexity of associations giving rise to a myriad of choices in its actions. And yet the responses are mechanical: the strength of the stimulus largely dictates which pathway of action is chosen, and if there is a conflict, it lasts but a brief moment. Choice, and the corresponding emotional states, present little conflict in the life of an animal. In a person, however, the operation of this associative process takes place within a number of constraints: I have to catch a bus by four o'clock if I don't want to miss my appointment; I must remember to buy some milk on my way home; there are messages on my answering machine I haven't listened to. We don't have simply a more complex mental field than animals; we also have more cognitive complexity—facts, beliefs, things that mean something. And for most of us, such knowledge *means* anxiety, desire, and fear.

For a young toddler, such concerns do not exist. A child—or at least a very young one—lives in the moment. While she is playing in the park, she doesn't worry about whether it will rain, about who is going to make dinner, about how the next mortgage payment is going to be met. But for an adult this *contextual* framework casts a constant shadow over our lives, creating a sense of oppression about getting things done, a fear of time moving too quickly. We have all had the experience of worrying about a letter we have to write, about the coming work week, about a problem we are having at work—all while putting out the garbage.

For humans, then, there is a complicated mental activity taking place all the time, within the context of emotional concern about the future. Young children are completely absorbed in the immediate present without concern for the future, but mature adult life demands that we constantly reflect and discriminate between possible goals and priorities. We have to direct our activities; we have to conform to the demands of the environment. And yet we are at the mercy of all sorts of trains of associations. For many adults, the complex mental world we live in is a battlefield, particularly when we consider the whole network of concerns that hover over us in the context of beliefs that often have an emotional impact on our every waking moment. In short, the field of consciousness is not only very active and busy; it is disturbed.

This explains why it is necessary for the mental field to quiet down. The field of consciousness needs to operate as a normal function. But because the ideo-motor mechanism is out of balance, this field becomes increasingly disturbed, especially in the face of the complications and difficulties imposed by adult life and concerns. This becomes clearer if you visualize ideo-motor action graphically. Ideas that discharge into motor acts constitute a vertical pathway. The various ideas that compete for discharge—the association of ideas—form a horizontal pathway. If the vertical pathway of ideo-motor action is sufficiently uncontrolled, producing a short-circuiting of motor acts, then this creates a horizontal disturbance of ideas, an association of ideas that constitutes a noisy mental field, or subconscious mental disturbance. (See Figure 8.) When the ideo-motor mechanism is restored to its normal working, then the overall level of vertical activity diminishes, and this in turn allows a cessation of the horizontal associative activity, or a quieting of the mental field.

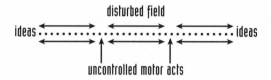

Figure 8
The disturbed field of consciousness

This shows why, and to what extent, the psychological dimension of ideo-motor action involves our emotional life. Any organism capable of spontaneous behavior is, neurologically speaking, complex, but the human organism is complex indeed, and this is what invests life with such emotional energy. We live, literally, in our heads; worry and fear subconsciously gnaw at us. When this activity ceases, we then become aware of this busy field—not in the sense of seeing it (that would mean we are on the outside looking in), but rather in the sense that we become aware of a quieting of preoccupation, a letting go of worry. We then feel as if a subliminal mental activity has ceased, as if we have suddenly woken up and found ourselves in a strange place: we see the walls, the room, hear sounds, as if they are new, as if we have just been transported into the sensory and perceptual reality of the present moment, free of thought and worry.

When this subconscious activity in the mental field quiets down, we then understand the calm and presence we must have felt as children. No one who has gazed into the eyes of a young child can fail to see how open, how alert, how free of tomorrow is the child that is unhindered by adult concerns. That gaze is the gaze of someone who lives in the moment, who is vital and aware of what is going on. In contrast, the adult is preoccupied, too distracted by inner fears and concerns to be fully aware

of the world around him. To regain that vital, youthful quality of alertness is to experience the awareness and detachment of a child, but at a
conscious level.

Understanding the relation of thinking to action explains why methods for heightening consciousness are so inadequate to deal with the problem. Since thought is connected not only to actual daily activities but to
the mechanism of activity itself, it is futile to address the problem of
quieting the mind by utilizing methods that bring about a relaxed state,
trance, hypnosis, and the like; the only solution is a heightened awareness of the process of activity itself.

Understanding the relation of thinking to action also explains how
emotional states of worry and nervous strain are connected with the
psychology of the unified working of mind and body. When we have
everyday worries, we usually think of them in terms of what causes them,
and in this sense consider them to be symptomatic of something subjective—some inner concern or issue. In fact, though, such emotional states
are secondary to the actual working of the ideo-motor system: when the
normal activity of the ideo-motor mechanism is restored, it has the effect
of quieting this mental disturbance.

We think, then, that emotions cause us to get worried. Sometimes,
however, getting worked up causes us to get worried, causes the mental
field to become disturbed, making us think and fret over the future.
The worry in this case is the result, not the cause, of the problem. The
solution is to calm down, in order for the field to quiet down, in order
to see things rationally again. That is why living calmly is an art, a discipline, not just a condition or problem to be treated. To find out why
one is worried, or to practice techniques for relaxing, is often futile,
because everyday worry, the stress of daily life, has no cause in the usual
psychological sense. The only solution is to take responsibility for one's
life, because it is the mode of living itself that causes the worry.

Deeper emotional problems, then, may stem from causes that do not
relate to activity as such. But it does not follow that basic, normal stress
or emotional states can be fathomed through introspection. When we suffer from worry, when we are in a "state," we are often aware of the specific content which causes that state. But we forget the relation of mind

to action. Neurotic activity—in the sense of states of worry and preoccupation—is usually thought to be a cause of physical distress, not a by-product of physical activity. But this sort of mental activity is neurotic by virtue of its relation to an imbalanced mechanism of activity. Even when the neurotic mental activity becomes a problem in and of itself, that problem is still a fact about the mind's relation to activity—in other words, about action itself.

The key to understanding the problem of mental balance, then, is conscious awareness in living. We may know how to live as animals, but we do not know how to live as humans, and we are not born knowing. Emotional states are dependent on how we conduct ourselves, not simply on whether we are aware of specific problems or issues. A truly balanced mental state can result only through mastery of the art of conscious control in living.

It is also important to realize that this change in mental activity is based not simply on the body but on motor function. By practicing relaxation, for instance, it is possible to achieve a kind of quieting down, to notice distracting thoughts, and to reduce stress. We saw earlier, however, that relaxing is often a form of collapsing, and as such, it represents a false attempt to restore the body to its normal condition. Relaxation doesn't restore muscle tension to a true state of balance, and as a result, the mental state also cannot become balanced. Even worse, relaxing will often complicate the subconscious activity associated with tension, not quiet it. Because ideo-motor action is subconscious, any process that causes preoccupation or abdication of consciousness can only complicate the reactions associated with it. By withdrawing from an active and alert condition, relaxation does just that: it dulls the awareness instead of heightening it.

The physical state that is associated with mental activity can be addressed properly only by restoring the body to a state of poise—that is, a relaxed but active state. Then and only then can the entire activity associated with the wrong working of the body quiet down fully. If, for instance, there is a condition of tension in the neck and back that is related to the activity of typing, establishing the muscle tone that is proper to normal activity makes it possible to perceive this underlying activity and, finally, to stop it; and this in turn demonstrates the relationship between subconscious mental activity and motor function.

The key to this change is the experience of stopping. If, through the practice of a relaxation method, one produces a calm state, it would not be possible to draw the connection between ideas and motor activity; we would instead make the vague observation that reducing tension in the body lowers the level of stress. When one restores the body to a state of balance and poise, however, one becomes suddenly aware of the mind quieting down as a direct result of a cessation of motor activity. There is a sense of having been subliminally doing things, subconsciously working on a problem or fretting over the coming work week, and all of a sudden this activity has stopped. This realization that some underlying activity has ceased—not just mentally but in fact—demonstrates in a startling way the direct link between ideas and muscular activity. Mental activity is not a vague state of mind, but the field of consciousness as it functions in relation to motor activity.

This explains why the problem of ideo-motor action intimately involves our emotional life. The problem of living well—of living sanely and calmly—is a problem involving this field; and this field, in turn, reflects how we actually conduct ourselves. The working of this field, in other words, does not somehow vaguely correspond to emotions but to the problem of living itself, and it manifests, when we are unable to live calmly, in the form of uncontrolled reaction. This explains why this field of consciousness—this complex psychological process—has an emotional aspect. We literally are struggling to live, and this aspect of our psychology— this field of consciousness as it functions as the psychological aspect of our actual reactions in living—is the stage where this drama is being enacted, both during waking hours and during sleep.

It is important to remember, though, as I mentioned in the discussion of reaction, that we are speaking of a specific aspect of psychology. Developmental psychology has tended to explain human behavior in terms of underlying motivations and relationships that are essential to the emotional well-being of a growing child or of the mature adult; and because we have not yet conceived of a psychological concept of how mind and body work as a unified organism, it is too often assumed that emotional states emanate from these deeper causes. As I've said, however, basic emotional states of worry and stress in fact belong more properly to the domain of everyday conduct—namely, the working of the unified mental and physical system in activity. In other words, everyday worry and stress must be understood from the point of view of a normal concept of how the mind and body function in everyday living.

But to explain away all emotional problems on the basis of the concept of mind/body unity discussed here is an equally dogmatic assertion. States of outright emotional disturbance are traceable to upbringing, chemical imbalances, and other developmental and situational issues that fall within the domain of psychopathology. Normal states of worry or concern are just that—normal, and must be clearly distinguished from emotional disturbance, affective disorders, addictive problems, and emotional disturbance *per se*—all of which fall under another category entirely. These latter problems are not caused by the wrong working of mind and body as a functional system, and cannot be adequately treated by becoming aware of one's actions and reactions. In other words, we must distinguish between "normal" disturbance and neurotic or pathological disturbance. The discipline of conscious awareness and control must be pursued for the right reasons and utilized in its proper context.

Conscious Control

All along I have insisted that the problem of stress and tension can be addressed only through the practice of conscious awareness and control applied to the organism in action. This demands that we conceive of mind and body as a unified whole, and apply our understanding of this unity to the fundamental educational question of how to raise the process of activity to a conscious level. I would like to turn finally to the problem of conscious control.

In the last section, I said that, when Richard sits down to work at a computer keyboard, he is not able to prevent the pattern of habitual tension because, once he actually begins the process of typing, he invokes the usual ideo-motor response. We saw that this response is further complicated by the complex network of associations that occur subconsciously and which constitute a kind of constant inner activity. By learning to stop,

Richard was able to bring about a balanced physical and mental activity associated with lowered stress. This also brought about a heightening of conscious awareness, and a quieting of the disturbed mental field.

This change, however, doesn't mean that Richard can now prevent the harmful pattern of tension when he actually performs an action in the context of daily life. When he now tries to type, at the moment he raises his arm to the keyboard, the tendency to react in the old harmful way, as well as the tension itself, will certainly be reduced. But the act of typing, because it makes Richard think about typing, will continue to initiate the wrong activity associated with the old pattern. The idea will still operate against his will; the problem will recur each time he actually faces the task of typing.

It is necessary, in order for him to solve the problem, to find a way of performing the action without actually thinking of doing it, and he must of course achieve this result without outside help. Earlier, for instance, we saw that when the teacher could ask him to perform certain simple actions that did not associate with the finished act, Richard could in this way complete the total act without ever having invoked the usual ideomotor pattern. The key to the problem was to focus entirely on the process, and in this way avoid thinking of the act itself.

In real-life activities, though, this is far more difficult than it appears. We saw, earlier, that action is meant to be subconscious, and this makes it difficult to perceive. Even when we choose to do something, we are meant not to have to think about it; this is the meaning, the very reality, of how action evolved. Although Richard can consciously choose to do the action or refrain from doing it, the thought process underlying the action—and in fact the entire act—remains largely automatic and -instinctive.

Trying to circumvent the idea that elicits these actions is also, as we've seen, extremely difficult. It is possible, for instance, to momentarily think of something else, and in this way avoid the pattern of tension associated with typing. But once Richard actually engages in the act of typing, once he thinks about what words he wants to type, the subconscious process associated with typing is brought into play, and he finds that, in spite of his intention to maintain the improved state, he has reverted to his usual harmful condition.

The improvement in coordination, though, provides a standard by which to actually observe the pattern happen, and this is the beginning of a solution. As the muscular tone in the back and neck is restored to a normal level, this provides a ground against which, when the idea comes to act, the old pattern can be perceived. This kinesthetic background provides the basis for raising the normally subconscious process to a conscious level. At an earlier stage of the process, Richard could kinesthetically perceive an increase in tension when he initiated an action; this was the beginning of raising the subconscious process to a conscious level. But kinesthetically sensing the reaction didn't make it possible to perceive how he himself subconsciously initiated that action by thinking of typing and thus triggering the action. Now that he is observing, and taking full responsibility for, his own actions, he can begin to see that he is himself initiating the action as a result of his own subconscious decision to type. The kinesthetic awareness now becomes the background for perceiving this subconscious process. At the moment he thinks of typing, he can perceive the mechanical train of thought, the idea, that actually triggers the action. He finally has full control over the process because it is now conscious.

At first, the ability to perform the action of typing without interfering with this system is sporadic. At the moment he acts, Richard finds that he has interfered and, in spite of himself, has reverted to the pattern. But as he develops a clearer perception of when the pattern of tension begins, he can strengthen his resolve to stick more firmly with the intention not to interfere with the system, making it possible to raise the arm and hit the key, but without the usual interference associated with his usual idea of typing.

This proves to be the key to the problem. Earlier, I said that the muscular system had an innate, or reflexive, design, and that the harmful pattern of tension interfered with it. Until now, Richard could prevent the pattern of tension sufficiently to bring about the reflex working of this system, but once he actually performed actions on his own, he interfered in some unconscious way. Because he can now command a conscious use of the system, he can notice the pattern that interferes with it and, in so doing, consciously prevent it. Richard now finds that he can perform the action in an almost effortless manner, with the result that the system can now work unimpeded.

Preventing the ideo-motor pattern at this conscious level makes it possible, finally, to fully remove the interference in the working of the system. We have seen, throughout this book, that there is a pattern of tension that interferes with the natural working of the muscular system, and that it occurs as part of the pattern of voluntary activity and is for this reason difficult to prevent. We are not normally aware of the extent to which the system is designed to operate in a reflexive or automatic way, nor of the extent to which the natural muscular system has become compromised over time as a result. By observing the pattern of tension in the teaching situation, we were able to remove some of this interference and to restore a coordinated working of the system, thus demonstrating that what appeared to be a specific problem was really part of a total pattern of interference. Up until now, Richard has been able to restore this pattern with the help of a teacher, and by becoming aware of the ideo-motor pattern, he was able to identify the cause of the interference.

The true context of ideo-motor action, however, is everyday life, and this means that the underlying source of this interference—namely, what Richard does in everyday life—is still virtually unchanged. We saw, for instance, that Richard had a tendency to shorten and constrict the back, and when we stopped this pattern in the controlled teaching situation his back was allowed to function more or less normally. This process, however, does not fully restore the healthy condition of the back because the ideo-motor pattern operates subconsciously during his daily activities, and this subconscious influence is far more widespread than the relatively short-term effect of preventing the habits during the teaching situation. The true source of the problem—namely, what he does during voluntary action—is still outside his field of awareness, and is therefore unchanged.

Now, however, Richard is preventing the harmful subconscious activity at its source, with the result that, for the first time, the underlying interference with this system is fully removed. As a result, the normal reflex response of the muscular system against gravity—the capacity of the muscular system to lengthen and expand in response to gravity—is allowed fully to work. There is a spontaneous and natural lengthening and improvement in muscle tone throughout the torso, an improvement in breathing, and an overall increase in vitality. The overall response that before had been so easily triggered by the idea of actions to be performed has now ceased, resulting in a quieting of the system, removal of tension and unnecessary activity, and a disappearance of the symptoms associated with this harmful activity.

Consciously preventing the pattern of habitual activity that interferes with the natural working of the system represents the true key to the problem that has impeded our progress at every stage. I've said all along that motor acts are not willed, but issue "upon the mere thought of it." We've been able to observe this reality, perhaps most graphically, when we trigger someone into an activity such as jumping out of a chair, and reveal how action is linked with subconscious associations. But this pattern normally works during voluntary action, and this means that to truly solve the problem, it must be addressed in the context of Richard's own activities, and through his own initiative. Until now, this was virtually impossible because, although Richard could perceive changes in tension, as well as the improved working of the physical system, he had no way of perceiving the subconscious activity of the ideo-motor system itself.

Now that he is able to see what he is doing in activity, however, he is preventing this subconscious pattern at its source—namely, during voluntary activity. And this is possible because he is now conscious of the process—that is, he has raised the normally subconscious activity of the ideo-motor system to a conscious level. Only when the system is sufficiently balanced does it then become possible, against the background of this heightened kinesthetic awareness, to perceive the normally subconscious operation of the idea, and to prevent this activity. When coordination improves to the point that the mental field is quiet and there is a state of heightened awareness, this increased sensory awareness makes it possible to perceive the subconscious pattern of activity and to replace it with an act consciously performed.

Becoming aware of mental activity that normally operates at a sub-conscious level raises mental functioning to the conscious plane. We saw earlier that ideas that lead to action do not occur singly, but in the context of a complex and neurotic field of ideas competing for discharge. It may be possible, in the context of this disturbed mental activity, to detect the physical aspect of a response, but the idea that triggers it is indistinguishable among the many ideas competing for discharge within this noisy field. When this field becomes quiet, however, it is then possible, against the now quiet mental background, to see the idea that triggers an action. The normally subconscious process of thought is now raised to a conscious level.

Perceiving the subconscious activity that triggers action leads to a more balanced mental activity. In the last several chapters we saw that reaction is associated with disturbance, worry, and preoccupation, which in turn create a disturbed mental field of activity. By stopping and allowing the system to return to a calm state, this mental field was able to quiet down, resulting in a more alert, balanced state of mind. The source of this mental activity, however, is the idea as it actually functions in activity, and until the ideo-motor response has become conscious and can be prevented, the subconscious associations that trigger action will continue to disturb this mental field. When the pattern itself is perceived, however, this makes it possible not simply to quiet the mind but to recognize the operation of ideas that fuel this associative activity. The mind not only becomes free of the usual neurotic disturbance, but the underlying subconscious activity—the true source of this disturbance—is now removed.

This perception of subconscious mental activity also has the effect of heightening mental awareness. In the last section we saw that the ideas that give rise to actions are not subconscious in the sense of being repressed or buried from awareness; "subconsciousness" simply refers to the instinctive, or habitual, operation of activity in humans and animals. When the mental field is quiet, and we then perceive the subconscious ideas that give rise to actions, however, we are, in essence, raising this subconscious process to a conscious level. In this sense we are not only becoming aware of a harmful pattern of response but illuminating that part of the mind which operates subconsciously, making it possible to then perceive the play of ideas in the mental field as they actually occur. The mind is now awakened, or conscious, because the thought process that is normally hidden from awareness is now revealed. It is then possible to observe ideas that give rise to fear and worry and that operate habitually as part of the subconscious pattern. By making this process conscious, the habitual operation of thought is extinguished, burning away constellations of neurotic activity, and leaving in their place a heightened consciousness and an awakened mind.

Raising the operation of ideas to a conscious plane implies a new level of balance in action and living. We all seek calmness and control in action in specific ways that allow us to behave more rationally, to observe and think clearly, to perform skilled feats, or to enhance aesthetic and spiritual awareness. But since our actions occur at a mainly subconscious level, this ideal is imperfectly achieved for the most part. In spite of being relatively calm at times, or attempting to relax and heighten our awareness, the mental field is more or less disturbed by subconscious activity at all times, in keeping with how we actually live day to day. When we actually engage in activity, the psychophysical process governing our actions is largely subconscious and, over time, susceptible to disturbance, loss of control, and imbalance. But this subconscious process can, through the process of coordinating the body and perceiving responses that link with ideas, become available to consciousness. By raising the level of awareness, the process is thus brought under control, rendering it less susceptible to deterioration over time, as well as available to readjustment and reeducation if deterioration or loss of control have occurred. It raises the subconscious process itself to a conscious level, bringing action and reaction under conscious control in every phase of life.

We have now traced the problem from our initial observations of the pattern of bodily tension to its fundamental source in the subconscious working of the system. In the previous discussion on behavior and reaction, I observed that in the field of psychology we typically regard physical symptoms as manifestations of underlying mental or emotional causes; we do not normally regard mundane acts as significant in themselves. We have now arrived, through a study of physical action, at a higher level of functioning and conscious awareness. In our culture, we often regard action as a means to an end; the physical acts of living and the "body" that carries them out are not valued as things in themselves. But the study of action has led us, first, to an understanding of the coordinated working of the muscular system, then to an understanding of the relation of this physical system to activity, and finally to a mode of conscious activity that makes it possible to perform actions in such a way as to prevent the interference with this system. All along, we have identified the problem not simply as a condition to be treated but as a pattern of activity arising from our subconscious functioning. In previous chapters, we observed how physical symptoms are linked with the working of the entire body in movement. We then saw how this physical pattern of tension, in turn, is linked with activity. Finally, we saw how this activity is associated with disturbance and stress. Each of these elements clearly shows that methods designed to treat symptoms of stress and tension do not, in fact, address the cause of these problems, because they fail to identify the behavioral and psychophysical dimension of the problem.

But no factor is more important to fully appreciating the significance of these factors than the element of consciousness. When we suffer from a symptom—particularly when it is chronic or debilitating—we often become convinced that there is something wrong with us, something physically defective. Even when we embrace the idea that the mind can cure the body or that we need to treat the person holistically, the view that the mind can heal the body presupposes that there is, in fact, something wrong that has to be cured. We are, in other words, culturally imbued with the concept that ill health must be cured by relying on some form of treatment or cure; the recent holistic theories about mind and body are no exception. Even when we recognize, as we have done in the last several chapters, that particular kinds of problems can be eradicated by removing the pattern of tension that interferes with the coordinated working of the body, and that this pattern of tension corresponds to our own actions, we resist the notion that we are ourselves responsible for the problem and that, in many cases, there is in fact nothing physically wrong with us.

When we can identify what we are doing in activity to interfere with the muscular system, and consciously prevent that interference from taking place, we are oriented to the problem in a completely new way. The physical system, we saw, is designed to reflexively maintain a balanced pattern of muscle tension. When the working of this system is compromised, it is mainly because of what we are doing in activity to interfere with it. If a symptom is associated with the interference in this system, it will disappear once the interference is removed. We may be convinced that some part of the body is injured or in need of treatment, but the problem in fact emanates from how we are using the system in activity— that is, from our own actions—and thus the true cause of the problem is our own subconscious activity. In short, there was nothing wrong, except the harmful pattern of subconscious activity that created the problem, and the only real solution is to consciously recognize and prevent this activity.

Identifying the role of consciousness is therefore crucial to fully understanding and solving the problems we've addressed in this book. It is possible, in attempting theoretically to make sense of this field, to stop at any point we have described in the course of these discussions and derive all sorts of practical applications based on one or another aspect. Many therapeutic techniques for relieving muscular strain and reducing stress have been developed, based solely on principles of physical functioning. It is also possible, at a more sophisticated level, to derive enormous benefit from learning to calm down, or by learning to become conscious of physical tension and strain during movement. But such derivations are specious if used as the basis for a complete theory. The key elements in understanding the problem of stress associated with daily living are the coordinated working of the entire body and its relation to subconscious ideas in action. Learning to consciously prevent this subconscious activity is the primary problem that must be faced in order to address the cause of tension and stress. The capacity to consciously recognize the pattern of action, although it occurs at the end of this discussion, is primary to correctly framing all the issues that led up to this point in our study.

This central role of consciousness also places therapeutic benefits in proper perspective. Because problems are perceived as physical, it is easy for many people to assume that physical improvements hold the key to solving whatever symptoms are causing discomfort. But without the capacity for conscious control, physical changes, however dramatic, will be relatively meaningless. As we've seen, the true purpose of the physical changes we've discussed early in the book is to facilitate one's awareness and control in action. When, therefore, bodily coordination is improved, its ultimate purpose is not to treat the physical symptom or even to correct the imbalances in the overall muscular system (although this latter element is crucial), but to provide a sensory criterion that makes it possible to gain control over the underlying faulty action that causes it. Such a process opens up the possibility of perceiving, and therefore gaining control over, the subconscious activity that is responsible for the malcoordination in the first place—a process that goes far beyond therapy and enters the domain of education.

Important as they are, then, changes made at the physical level are not the goal, but a means to a larger end. In this sense, all the prior stages that we have looked at—restoring the physical system to its proper working, observing and learning to prevent the ideo-motor response in simple actions such as sitting or standing, quieting the reactions associated with the wrong working of this system—are only preparations for the most fundamental stage of the process—namely, conscious control in action. Such re-educational work is often required in order to deal with the complications that impede the natural working of the postural system and the coordinated working of the body. But to derive a clinical theory based on the benefits of such work misleads one into thinking that the true context of these discoveries is clinical when in fact it is educational. If the symptom is ultimately caused by the subject's own subconscious activity, then the problem isn't with the body but with the subject's own behavior, and only the subject can take full responsibility for that problem—a challenge that is educational in the truest sense of the word.

The central role of consciousness also reveals why awareness alone isn't sufficient to solve the problems dealt with in this book. Early in our discussion, we saw that it was necessary to reduce tensions that were part of an observable pattern of movement. But noticing such tension, even during activity, failed to solve the problem completely because the tension was itself initiated as part of the total activity. Only when the overall system was consciously restored to its proper working was it possible to recognize, and prevent, the pattern of interference as a response pattern. This process, we saw, was based on a consciousness of the total pathway of activity, and therefore involved an awareness not simply of muscles but of a total subconscious pattern of response that must be consciously perceived to be stopped.

Methods designed to help the subject become aware of the body in movement and at rest, then, do not address the underlying problem, in spite of appearances to the contrary. To try to be aware during activity is a contradiction in terms, since all activity is initiated by a subconscious process that, by definition, invokes the very harmful habits one is trying to prevent. Only when tension is conceived not simply in relation to movement but as part of the total pathway of activity is it possible to prevent it. Ultimately, the problem of misdirected action cannot be solved by attention to the body alone, but only by learning to recognize and gain conscious command of the pattern of activity itself.

This element of consciousness reveals what is perhaps the fundamental cause of the problems we've looked at in this book. In our inquiry, we have identified a number of crucial factors contributing to tension and strain. The pattern of tension that interferes with the innate working of the muscular system; the relation of muscular tension to a total pattern of activity; the harmful levels of reaction and stress that develop as a result of the lowered standard of the functioning of this pattern of activity— all are important elements in understanding the problem of the control of stress. But when we identify the role of consciousness in ultimately solving the problem, we then have a new and far more elevated description of causality—namely, the fact of our activity being subconscious. There has been much speculation about whether humankind is inherently degenerate, structurally faulty, and unusually prone to disease; certainly there is truth in such speculation. But perhaps no single explanation for the physical degeneration of humankind is more compelling than the simple fact that when faced with the various tasks of civilized life, most people are simply ill-equipped to function efficiently or to maintain their natural poise. In this sense, there is nothing wrong with us except the fact that we must live under civilized conditions, and no solution except to learn to bring the body, and our use of it in the various activities of daily life, under conscious control. We must command, in our civilized life, not only a more sophisticated use of tools and technology, but must also evolve to a more sophisticated control and use of ourselves.

This evolutionary context reveals what is, in the final analysis, the crucial challenge in the control of stress. It is tempting, when examining the origins of problems relating to health, to be biased in favor of treatments and methods that produce immediate empirical results, and even to subordinate consciousness to its role in alleviating physical symptoms. But our inquiry has ultimately led beyond issues of health and faulty conditions in living to the broader question of the control of behavior itself. If the harmful conditions we have observed are connected with a subconscious process of activity, then the solution to the problem is to raise the process governing these conditions to the conscious plane.

This central role of consciousness is also critical to understanding the problem from the point of view of development. We observed in the earlier chapters that children, at an early age, usually exhibit a high level of functioning—so much so that, in many ways, they exemplify the conditions we are seeking in health and functioning, at both a mental and physical level. With time, however, the child's innate physical poise is lost. Coordination deteriorates, physical vitality is lowered, and actions and reactions become increasingly uncontrolled, leading to disturbance and stress. This means that however desirable the conditions of childhood may appear, the child lacks the one crucial element that it needs to maintain those conditions: consciousness of how he or she functions. The child is ultimately robbed of health and balance by his or her own subconscious activity.

Children, then, may be better balanced than adults at this early stage in their lives; they may be free of overall mental disturbance and physical degeneration. But their action is nevertheless subconscious, and it is this fact which ultimately leads to deterioration in even the healthiest of children. It is therefore useless to romanticize the conditions of childhood or the promise of a return to a more primitive state. We are again led to the conclusion that if we are to solve the problem of stress and strain, it is necessary, ultimately, to elevate the process underlying these conditions to a conscious level.

A New Field for Prevention

In the beginning of this book, I pointed out that a class of problems has emerged that falls not within medicine or psychology, but within an area that is generally defined as mind and body. In response to the demand to solve these problems, a new paradigm in health and the study of mind and body has emerged, characterized by various techniques that demonstrate the subtle interdependence of mind and body. It has been my contention, however, that these methods do not fully address the question of what is causing these symptoms, and so represent an inadequate attempt at articulating a field that, as yet, has been only partially understood. When we perceive how the body works as a system, its relation to activity, and how we can raise the process to a conscious level, in so doing we conceive the subject in practical terms that address not simply how to improve the system, but what the problem is and how to unravel its fundamental causes. This subject of ideo-motor action represents an area of psychology that recognizes mind and body as a functional whole, and that utilizes this knowledge toward a practical understanding of action and how to bring it under conscious control.

The first element in this subject, as we've seen, is a practical or functional concept of physiology as it relates to action and movement. There is an extensive literature in the mind/body field that demonstrates the empirical effects of various relaxation techniques in reducing muscular tension and stress and raising immune function, but which fails to articulate what is actually wrong with the body and why. We addressed this problem in a practical way by observing how the muscular system works in movement, what we do to interfere with it, and how harmful patterns of tension interfere with functioning—in short, how the postural system works and what's wrong with it.

But physiology alone, as we've seen, isn't sufficient to make sense of the problem of stress and tension. Even when the physical system is balanced, any involvement in action will evoke the ideo-motor response, and therefore bring about precisely those factors that interfere with this balance. Introducing this element makes it possible to uncover the mental element in activity and, in turn, its connection with patterns of action and reaction that must be raised to a conscious level in order to remove the interference in the physical system.

Together, these two elements comprise the outlines of what is, essentially, a new field—the mind and body viewed as one system of functional activity. In the emerging mind/body field, the most common way of expressing the link of mind and body is to amalgamate physiology and psychology into an interactionist concept of a mental force whose empirical effects on the body can be identified and described. But because such descriptions do not take into account the actual subconscious operation of the system in activity, it is necessary to gain a knowledge of the functioning whole that integrates both physiological knowledge and psychology into a functional whole, and that embodies a practical understanding of behavior as it relates to the physiology of muscle tension and action.

At the heart of this concept is a unified view of mind and body that goes beyond the notion of mind and body as connected systems. Many people recognize that symptoms of stress do not represent medical problem as such; stress is seen to involve a subtle interplay of mind and body and therefore cannot be treated as a purely medical problem. But the true significance of the mind/body connection, as we've observed it, is not simply that the mind and body are linked, but that the link signifies a subconscious pattern of activity that occurs in normal activity and that must be raised to a conscious level in order to prevent this wrong activity. Methods for influencing the body through the mind may produce therapeutic results, and by appealing to the link between mind and body, they may appear to be more enlightened than traditional medical approaches. But because these methods don't address the actual problem—namely, the operation of the organism in activity as a behavioral unity—they exploit the notion of a mind/body connection, while leaving our true potential—and the possibilities this opens up for improved functioning and health—completely untapped. In theoretical terms, the interactionist concept of mind and body mystifies the exact relation of mind and body, and uses the mystery itself as part of the lure and appeal of techniques that are employed to bring about therapeutic changes. In short, it elevates the lack of clarity to a category of understanding.

The very claim that the mind affects the body, then, is dualistic, and it hinders progress in exploring the mind and body precisely by creating the illusion that such a concept adequately addresses the problem of stress, when in fact it deals only with symptoms. Once we conceive of the fundamental problem of activity as a total pathway that must be brought to consciousness, we can integrate knowledge in the physiological domain not simply in order to legitimize methods on the basis of their therapeutic effectiveness, but to create a truly educational approach to stress. This concept represents a true psychology of mind and body based on a solid foundation of practical and theoretical knowledge.

This concept of mind/body unity is unique also to the field of psychology, for a number of reasons. First, in this century, psychology has been informed by a physiological concept of action and function that conceives mind and body as a unified whole—as in the study of perception and motor learning. But this knowledge, when it isn't purely descriptive, is conceived largely in medical and experimental terms and has little applicability to the practical problems of living itself. What is required is a physiology of the use and functioning of the organism in activity. This demands, in turn, a practical understanding of muscular activity and its relation to reaction.

Second, Western psychology has been so dominated by genetic and developmental explanations of behavior that it has all but ignored the potential for conscious development and control. Tension and stress, for instance, are still largely viewed as caused by outside factors; when we say mind affects body, what we mean in practice is that our response to outside stresses (mental) causes bodily harm (physical). Accordingly, most methods for treating stress offer a means of recovering from or reversing the effects of stress, but fail to empower the individual to rise above such adverse reactions. Stress-reducing methods for raising consciousness pay lip service to an educational ideal, but in practice they presume that outside forces have power over us and that we are therefore powerless to rise above these outside forces. The true problem is not how to clinically recover from the effects of stress—however useful that may be in a therapeutic context—but to realize our own potential to overcome the instinctive reactions that bring it about in the first place.

Third, psychology as a field has become continuous with physiologi-cal knowledge that conceives all mental phenomena as having a physical counterpart. The body itself, however, has little importance to such work. (Even the concept of ideo-motor action is used, in the work of William James, as part of a debate over the role of will in behavior; the body plays little role in this conception.) In developmental psychology the body is usually seen as an expression of mental or emotional states, or else has no place at all. As a field, psychology leaves out the mental ele-ments in action and the body in mental functioning; concern for bodily health is largely reserved for physical educators. But as we've seen, the pattern of bodily tension isn't incidental to behavior, but part of the uni-fied pattern of behavior itself. When viewed in this way, the body must be seen not as incidental to psychology but as an essential component in a functional psychology that is based on an appreciation of bodily func-tioning and its role in human behavior.

When seen in this way, the body can assume a more respected role as a subject worthy of study and an aspect of life deserving our personal attention. Our tendencies toward an introspective psychology—and per-haps our Western heritage as a whole, which tends to devalue the body—make it easy to minimize the significance of bodily function in living. Does it really matter that I tense my neck and back when I write at a desk? Do my physical actions really matter to the quality of my life? The answer is that our reactions, our mental attitude in living, our level of stress in living our daily lives, the very fabric of our conduct, are depen-dent on bodily functioning. The body is crucial to the quality of life itself, which is lived in the immediate present and whose value is con-tained in, among other things, simple actions and experiences. These sim-ple actions cease to be enjoyable and edifying in those who have succumbed to a reactive and harmful condition of functioning, but are enlightening to those who gain an appreciation for this aspect of living. The body is thus important, not simply because it is the basis for alter-ing wrong body patterns that affect us physically, or because the fate of our mental lives is theoretically or philosophically intertwined with phys-iology; it is central to the entire practical issue of stress and behavior in daily living, and to the capacity to live fully in the present moment.

Fourth, it is easy to assume that, because tension often has an emotional component, this emotional content holds the key to why we become tense to begin with. But no amount of introspection, psychological insight, or emotional clarity can solve the tensions a violinist suffers from while playing violin, or the throat problems that result from faulty or uncontrolled speech, for the simple reason that such problems are fundamentally linked with activity. Addressing these activities must involve changing emotional attitudes associated with such behaviors. But to deal successfully with this problem, it must be understood as a functional problem that is educational, not therapeutic, in nature.

Such a functional psychology of action sees behavior not as a manifestation of some underlying problem but as the problem itself. In modern introspective psychology, behavior is so often seen as the result of underlying motives or emotions that we automatically assume that physical symptoms are the expression of emotions, not that action itself is the problem. But we are designed for behavior, for doing things; it should not be surprising that how we do things itself comprises a unique branch of study, replete with its own psychological characteristics and problems.

The same is true of particular kinds of emotional states that, notwithstanding their psychic content, are not pathological or developmental in nature. As I pointed out a few moments ago, we normally think emotions cause us to get worried; but sometimes getting worked up causes us to get worried by disturbing the mental field. The emotional element in this case is the result, not the cause, of the problem. The solution is to restore physical and mental balance in order to see things rationally again. That is why living calmly is an art, a discipline, not just a condition to be treated. Introspective attempts to find the cause of this aspect of stress are beside the point, because the cause is directly related to behavior itself. The solution is not in methods that can solve the problem, but in our own capacity to take responsibility for our own conduct.

Yet if analysis of emotional content cannot solve the problems addressed in this field, it is equally important to acknowledge that addressing the ideo-motor problem is equally futile as a means of treating emotional problems. If the mental field, which is associated with various emotional states, becomes quiet as a result of conscious awareness and control, this in some sense transcends and even illuminates mental content. At the same time, however, it is important to recognize that such awareness cannot be sought as a means of dealing with emotional problems, or stress that stems from predominantly emotional causes. The problems we are dealing with are not essentially emotional but relate specifically to the functioning of the system in activity. The process of examining this aspect of functioning leads to an eradication of certain emotional states that belong, properly speaking, to the area of mind and body as a functional system. But such a process cannot substitute for treatment of pathological conditions or emotional problems that emanate from a fundamentally different source.

This distinction may seem, to those who prefer systems that combine the treatment of emotion, bodily states, and stress into one set of exercises or prescriptions, to fall short of a truly unified concept of mind and body. But the mind/body field is in fact a large and complex subject, and progress in this field depends more on precise knowledge than on ideological amalgamation and eclecticism. Perhaps because of a tendency to view physical symptoms as manifestations of emotions, or perhaps because of the apparent connection of such problems with stress, it is easy to subsume the subject of back pain and other everyday complaints within psychology as a whole. But we can no more hope to solve back trouble by considering it a function of psychology or medicine than we can learn to sing by studying physiology. We must recognize that the problems dealt with in this book have a practical nature, and as such must be studied in a practical way. The first criteria we must apply in arriving at an understanding of the causes of back trouble is to assess whether we are able to solve the problem. Without such practical solutions, no real progress can be made, however elaborate or impressive the theory.

My purpose, then, in advancing the ideas set forth in this book is not to diminish or deny the validity of other areas of psychology that view the family structure, genetics, or development as crucial to the study of various stress disorders, or to subsume such problems within an umbrella concept of psychophysical unity. The notion that all things psychic are somatic and *vice versa* is philosophically true. But when *a priori* truths and holistic ideologies are substituted for practical experience in learning how to intelligently identify and address particular kinds of problems, such truths become more dogmatic than insightful. My main concern is to address a specific type of problem that, as far as I have been able to determine, does not fall within existing areas of medicine or psychology as they are currently practiced, and which therefore must be defined as a new branch of psychology. Bodily tension and stress, insofar as they occur as an everyday problem that must be addressed as a matter of physical and mental control, are fundamentally related to the study of action. This function, insofar as it involves complex mental operations in relation to motor function, represents a new branch of psychology that, when applied in individual cases, falls within the field not of treatments or therapies but of education. This field—however much it may be necessary in practice to combine it with other techniques and insights—must be clearly articulated in its own right, and based on observation and insight into actual problems and clear insight into what steps must be taken in order to solve them.

At the other extreme, the pressure to empirically verify the benefits of mind/body techniques has led to a narrow behaviorism that is not sufficiently sensitive to the psychological aspects of how we function. Empirical tests of the effects of meditating, for instance, may in some sense prove the existence of a mental factor in treatment of stress or demonstrate the therapeutic benefits of consciousness. But by focusing on immediate and measurable therapeutic benefits, this approach shifts attention away from self-responsibility and insight and thus undermines the very concept of consciousness. Such techniques are clearly therapeutically useful, but as mind/body theories they are severely biased, for two reasons. First, producing measurable results, as we've observed throughout this book, may appear to demonstrate the existence of a mind/body connection, but by utilizing a behavioral technique, it circumvents the true element of conscious control that must be at the root of such a process. Second, producing a measurable effect does not in and of itself prove that the problem is being addressed. Any number of activities—contact with animals, human touch, sports, massage, aesthetic experience, listening to music, swimming, walking outdoors—measurably reduce the effects of stress; but such empirical results do not constitute a true solution to the problem of stress. A true theory of stress—one that embodies a clear understanding of the mind-body connection—must not simply demonstrate that a particular technique is effective, but must adequately explain the cause of the problem, how it manifests in behavior, and how it must be altered. Even more important, it must empower the individual to take full control of that process as a matter of personal growth, rather than appeal to an inner force or a therapeutic technique that is applied simply as an antidote to a problem that is taken for granted.

The fact is, many of the techniques that utilize consciousness to produce therapeutic results do not take consciousness seriously except as a clinical tool for training a passive subject to respond differently to stimuli that produce stress. This tendency reflects an underlying skepticism in behaviorism and the empirical sciences concerning the relevance, and even the existence, of consciousness. But in spite of the tendency in empirical science to diminish the importance of consciousness and the role of the mind except when its effects can be empirically verified, mind can be easily studied and "seen," once we know how to look—a fact that holds true for psychodynamic theories as well, which explain behavior at another level.

This principle applies also to conditioning theories of stress, which are unnecessarily biased in the direction of what is crudely observable. Once we perceive the mental component in tension and stress, it is clear that identifying overt responses, and then invoking, or inventing, the mechanism of conditioning to explain them, is in fact an abstraction. There is no such mechanism of conditioning; it is merely one among many influences on behavior, and to favor this influence merely because it corresponds to overt behavior is to minimize the complexity and subtlety of animal, not to mention human, behavior. In fact, once we observe the reality of action as a complex mental and physical pathway—and the necessity of raising this process to a conscious level—it is clear that the concept of conditioning was inferred from incomplete facts and has no real appreciation for the complex psychophysiology of human activity—the true subconscious mechanism that governs learned behavior and of which overt behaviors are really a function.

The concept of a unified working of mind and body also reveals the limitations of methods that promote the role of awareness as a device for altering harmful conditions. Awareness—particularly in popular methods that employ various devices for relieving muscular tension or relaxation—is often conceived as a kind of light that can be shined on the body. By aiming our awareness on ourselves, it is possible to relax muscles, lower blood pressure, and quiet the mind. But awareness in and of itself can have only a limited impact on the body, for two reasons. First, in order to achieve true physical relaxation, it is first necessary to gain an appreciation of how the body works and what has gone wrong with it. Such an appreciation arises not from awareness alone but from a clear understanding, based on observation of how the body works in movement, of what we are doing in activity. This makes it possible to use one's awareness in a constructive way, not simply as a way of engaging in a process blindly without any real understanding of what the problem is and whether the changes being made are adequately addressing it. Second, awareness of the body alone cannot solve a problem that is fundamentally connected with behavior. The problem of tension must be clearly conceived not simply as a physical problem but as a total behavioral pattern that must be brought under conscious control.

Distinguishing the various levels of the problem also points up a critical difference between being aware and being conscious. It is possible to perceive tension in an accurate way, to calm down the system so that daily behavior will be affected, to maintain this sensitivity during activity—in other words, to be aware—and yet to have little or no control over one's own actions. Only when the underlying pattern of activity itself is perceived is the problem really addressed; at this stage, it is not tension but the whole act that is perceived. Achieving this level of control, however, involves not simply awareness but an appreciation of the psychophysical nature of the problem. When we focus our awareness, we are utilizing a potential, a capacity; but it has no meaning unless it is linked with the larger problem of which it is in fact part. Ultimately, it is necessary to become aware not only of the body, but of a total behavioral process that must be brought to consciousness.

Making this distinction between awareness of muscle tension and awareness of the pattern of muscular activity, as I have pointed out in pre-

vious chapters, is another way of identifying the truly mental and physical nature of the problem. If, as many theories claim, everyday tension
is "carried" from earlier trauma or emotional stress, it would be possible
to remove these tensions simply by focusing directly on them, or else by
releasing the emotional trauma with which they are associated. But tension, as we saw, is most commonly connected with movement and activity, and so is directly involved with activity and the psychophysical process
that governs action. For this reasons, methods that conceive the problem
in terms of changes to be made in the physical system, or of the connection of tensions with psychic holdings, may be useful in relieving certain
strains, but they are oversimplifying a complex subject. The problem of
tension and how it links with the brain is in fact a unique subject area
that has its own special requirements, and one that must be articulated
and conceived clearly if practice is to live up to theory.

More recently, some authors have advanced the notion that bodywork, because it promotes awareness and develops mental and physical
pathways in the brain, is in fact a psychophysical process. But while it is
true that massage therapy, bodywork, and other forms of body awareness involve psychophysical processes, it does not follow that such techniques appreciate fully the concept of mind/body unity. Even the crudest
exercise technique is in fact psychophysical, because every function, however dualistically conceived, is by definition psychophysical. But such "psychophysical" techniques are, practically speaking, bankrupt. Massaging
the body may in fact involve all kinds of psychophysical processes, but
this does not mean it addresses the true unity in action of body and
mind. The meaning of dualism is not that things are separate, but that
we separate mind and body in our understanding and in the corresponding practices which reflect that misunderstanding.

Another misconception is the belief that because consciousness influences the body, alterations in states of consciousness hold the key to health.
But we can no more become conscious of our actions by being aware than
we can become kind and generous by feeling more positive and concerned
about people. Thinking isn't merely an inner subjective force that, by
being properly utilized, will result in corresponding bodily changes—a
mind state that, when altered, results in a corresponding alteration in real-

ity. Thinking is concrete; it is what we are. I rush, I worry, I have fear—all these things are my thinking. To merely get myself in a different state is to postpone dealing with these problems, not to alter them.

It is not possible, then, to be conscious in a vacuum. Consciousness, meditating, awareness—if these are to be real—do not involve simply achieving a subjective state, but actually observing the fact of what one is, and in so doing, to take true responsibility for one's thoughts, conduct, and choices. That is why, in serious spiritual traditions, meditation is pursued not as a means for change, but as part of an overall discipline that includes observing and taking responsibility for all aspects of one's life. When seen in this way, what does thinking differently, as a means of changing negative thoughts, actually do? What means are offered by such methods for actually understanding consciousness in a truly meaningful way, except to provide a superficial means for feeling better? True consciousness must involve perception and responsibility for what one actually is—in this case, one's actual way of doing things, reacting, and conducting oneself. This isn't a matter simply of quieting the mind, recovering from stress, or providing momentary relief from tension, but of actually being conscious of what is normally subconscious based on an actual appreciation of what one is doing in activity.

Nor is the main purpose of consciousness to affect health. Invoking the power of consciousness to influence bodily functioning, a number of mind/body methods promote meditation as a means of heightening consciousness and tapping the true potential for health. In practice, however, these methods subjugate the entire question of spiritual evolution to health, and in this sense do not elevate the role of consciousness but demean it as a means to an end. At the most fundamental level, the issues addressed in this book are not about health but about the quality of life. To speak of altering consciousness as a means of directly affecting the body may appear to raise the subject of health to a higher spiritual plane, but what it is really doing is subjugating spirituality to the level of promising and promoting cures.

Many writers also speak of consciousness as a kind of force that can cure illness and create conditions of health. But, at least insofar as the present topic is concerned, this is to misunderstand the role of the mind in influencing the body. Consciousness does not make changes happen; by removing interference, it makes it possible for the body to naturally restore itself. Claiming that consciousness has the power to create conditions of health is not only inaccurate and irresponsible; it also leaves out any real explanation of how results are produced. In fact, we are naturally imbued with the inherent organizational structure that, when allowed to work, makes bodily changes happen; the function of consciousness is to remove the impediments to nature. In this sense, consciousness does not have some miraculous power to be tapped into like some power source or to be sought based on promises and unfounded hope.

Underlying this health-oriented focus on consciousness is the desire not to be intelligent about health but to be cured, to get results. If we feel better, we usually don't want to go further, or think more about it; after all is said and done, the desire to understand the problem is weaker than the desire to have gotten rid of what ails us. We are wedded to the notion that there is something wrong with us, and we want to explore the mind/body connection in order to find a cure.

But if, as many recent mind/body theories claim, health problems involve much larger issues of quality of life and personal evolution, then it is not enough to promise benefits to be gained, but to identify the larger causes that must be solved, independently of immediate health issues. Too often the opposite is the case. Many theories cannot identify what purpose consciousness has except in relation to sickness, as if consciousness were invented as a tool for reversing illness. All aspects of human life require understanding and positive growth; we seek greater understanding as a means of moving along this path, whether or not we have particular problems motivating that interest. In the context of the present subject, we have been led to look at how the body works in action because there are, initially, health issues that forced us to look at it. But the real issue—and the issue we have identified upon deeper study—is to understand the subconscious basis of our functioning; consciousness cannot have meaning except in relation to those aspects of our functioning that must be brought to consciousness. Once we identify the underlying problem as a pattern of subconscious behavior that can be solved only through conscious control, then it is clear that the problem requires not methods and treatments but self-responsibility and conscious development. To identify the problem as psychophysical is to say that the problem isn't really clinical in nature, but educational. It indicates the potential not simply to develop more effective methods of curing illness but to evolve to a higher stage of functioning.

But beyond articulating a field, beyond benefits to be gained, there is the reality of conscious control, won through the discipline of self-mastery. This entire analysis was based on the examination of a concrete problem that we have been attempting to solve by raising the subconscious activity underlying behavior to a conscious level. But what, after all, is this consciousness? We can speak of it in impressive terms, as if it were a kind of magical force that transforms the body and cures illness. In fact, as we've seen, each and every change that happens can be accounted for on the basis, finally, of inherent functions that had been interfered with; we are getting no more than what animals have—the mental alertness, the physical efficiency—except consciously: the miracle of health is nature's miracle, not a miracle of consciousness. The function of consciousness, in the end, is to restore something that was lost, not to give us something we never had.

The most crucial component in this process, however, is distinctly human and, in this sense, unique—namely, the ability to raise action to a conscious plane. In the last section I pointed out that actions arise from a complex field of ideas that operate at a subconscious level. When the activity in this field ceased, the overactivity was removed. But the operation of the ideas themselves was still subconscious; it was then necessary to perceive the play of ideas in this field as they actually occur, which constitutes a conscious plane of functioning. When we raise the operation of ideas to this conscious level, this unveils the mechanical nature of all our activity, the hidden operation of thought. When the field is quiet, it is then possible to perceive the ideas that trigger action, to unveil the mechanical operation of mind and body and, finally, to raise the process of action itself to a conscious plane. No method—however therapeutically beneficial—can address the actual source of the problem in the ongoing activity of the system or can substitute for becoming consciously aware of one's own activity.

This quality, this heightened awareness, is more than restoring something that we have lost, more even than having the freedom of movement, the stillness and quiet, of an animal. To be able to perceive the movement of thought is to have awakened the mind itself, and this mental awareness, achieved through stillness and non-doing, is among the highest arts of conscious self-mastery. Many mind/body practices frame progress in this realm in terms of emotional release and emotional awareness, as if the study of the body cannot be transcendent or spiritually fruitful except insofar as it aspires to personal insights leading to maturity and increased creativity or spontaneity. Certainly emotional health is important—so important, in fact, that it is a prerequisite for doing conscious work. But there are things in life higher than emotional balance— among them, the condition of stillness and heightened awareness in which mental content and personal emotions are transcended through insight arising from a quiet mind. There are many theories about this condition, and many methods that promise it, as if real insight can be achieved by blindly following a set of prescribed steps. But for those who aspire to real understanding, the true path is followed, in the end, through honest self-appraisal, humility, insight, and a willingness to come intimately to terms with the problem before trying to transcend it. This is the practical reality of conscious prevention and control, achieved through discipline and self-mastery: the realization of the transcendent inheritance of a conscious mind.

A Brief Historical Survey
of Mind/Body Techniques

At the beginning of this work, I briefly outlined some of the main trends in the study of mind and body. This brief synopsis, however, did not fully do justice to the extensive and varied methods that fall within these categories, or of their historical antecedents. The following literature review gives a bird's-eye view of this field and the various traditions which have contributed to it. This review is by no means exhaustive, but rather is intended to identify key works within an ever-growing mass of literature and to trace the philosophical and scientific origins of current practices. It should also be kept in mind that this literature review is not a review of methods for improving health, which would considerably expand its scope, but rather of techniques that deal, in a practical way, with the relationship of mind and body and with the practical concept of awareness or control applied in the context of this relationship.

Historical Overview

The subject of the mind and body in health is, as one might guess, broad indeed; but it is even broader than one first suspects. Even in the practice of medicine and healing that predates recorded history, it is clear that many shamans and healers both in the East and West had a wide appreciation of psychological factors that entered into health. From our knowledge of the school of Hippocrates (the "father of Western medicine"), it is clear that medical practice has always taken into account mental and psychological factors in healing. Even in our present highly specialized medical practices, the idea of the whole person (notwithstanding the recent development of a holistic movement which is challenging the mechanization and specialization in medicine) has remained intact in medical care in the doctor-patient relationship, in nursing, and in various cultural practices.

In a very general sense, then, healing practices have always recognized the interaction of mind and body, and to merely summarize the various practices associated with it could easily encompass several volumes and a span of many centuries, not to mention the many and diverse cultures throughout the world. But such an undertaking is not within the scope of this book, since my purpose here is to examine the mind/body subject as a practical topic of self-help, which limits the field considerably. Most practices relating to health, in fact, are not real mind/body practices and do not, in any real sense, practically address the problems we are speaking about here. So this further narrows the field.

But it is nevertheless worthwhile to mention the range of topics that might interest the reader who is exploring the historical antecedents of present-day mind/body theories. In the East, there is a wealth of traditions that could rightly be called mind/body practices, relating both to health and to martial arts and spiritual disciplines, many of which are practiced for their health benefits. In some cases, as in the martial arts, these involve a high degree of awareness and bodily control as well as spiritual discipline; spiritual disciplines also involve elements of awareness and bodily control that embrace implicit concepts of mind and body. Some of these practices—beneficial as they may be in addressing tension and stress—do not directly address the question of awareness but are intended either for combat or spiritual insight. Other techniques, such as Qi Gong and Tai Chi, are widely practiced precisely for the purpose of enhancing general health and well-being; I will briefly cover some of these practices as they are being taught today in connection with health, including Oriental medicine in general.

The Western spiritual tradition is not as rich as the East in mind/body disciplines *per se,* except perhaps in religious practices associated with early Christianity, which included contemplation and rigorous ascetic routines. There is a Western tradition of physical culture and martial development (modern exercise is partially derived from this source), but again, this isn't directly relevant to the subject of mind and body. Perhaps of more relevance are the many schools and practices of elocution, drama, dance, and movement training, which I will touch on briefly later.

The most prevalent mind/body practice in the Western world is to pursue mental and physical well-being by exercising each function separately, and by so doing to achieve a healthy whole. This Greek ideal of *mens sana in corpore sano*—a sound mind in a sound body—was articulated by Plato, who advocated education of mind and body: "Education has two branches," Plato wrote, "one of gymnastic, which is concerned with the body, and the other of music, which is designed for the improvement of the soul" (Plato, *Laws,* 7). This ideal of keeping physically fit is widely practiced today, and research on the effects of exercise have proven beyond doubt that exercise is not only physically beneficial but also improves alertness, performance, mental attitude, self-confidence, and general emotional health.

Perhaps of more general interest to this subject than the disciplines themselves is the tendency in the Western world (in contrast to the philosophy underlying Oriental medicine) to separate mind and body. Many people attribute the mind/body split, and the current trend toward a holistic perspective in health and healing, to the philosophical dualism of René Descartes. In fact, the dualism of mind and body in the Western world has older origins. Democritus, a pre-Socratic philosopher, emphasized the reality of the physical, material world, which is constructed of atoms (a view foreshadowing the reductionist tendencies of modern allopathic medicine); in contrast, Plato emphasized the immaterial world of "Forms"—the qualities common to various material objects such as color, or beauty—as the primary reality. In Plato's philosophy, the material world and the world of Forms were two distinct realms, and of the two the world of Forms was the more real (Jones 1952:103).

Descartes' philosophy, then, is certainly not the cause of the tendency in the Western world to separate mind and body; but his philosophy did bring this separation to fruition and, in so doing, heralded an era of mechanistic and specialized biology and medicine which characterize modern Western medicine. Descartes conceived mind and matter as two distinct substances—*res cogitans* and *res extensa*—that cannot act on one another. The body, which was an elaborate machine, in fact operated separately from the mind; the soul resides in the base of the brain, where it interacts with the body. There are therefore "two parallel but independent worlds, that of mind and that of matter, each of which can be studied without reference to the other" (Russell 1945:567). Thus the philosophy of Descartes "brought to completion, or very nearly to completion, the dualism of mind and matter that began with Plato and was developed, largely for religious reasons, by Christian philosophy" (567). This dualism is today reflected in the concept that mind and body are two distinct realms that interact; many of the current mind/body theories are attempts to bridge this gap.

Animal Magnetism, Hypnosis, and Suggestion

One of the most prevalent explanations underlying current methods for treating the causes of physical tension and stress is the view that unconscious or underlying emotions manifest in the form of psychosomatic symptoms. This conception of the role of mental and emotional factors in sickness and healing—both in Western and holistic medicine—owes its modern conceptual roots to the study of hypnotism and the subsequent study of the unconscious mind.

The phenomenon of hypnotism, and its graphic demonstration of the influence of mental phenomenon on the body, began with the work of Franz Anton Mesmer, an eighteenth-century physician. Influenced by occult thinkers of the fourteenth and fifteenth centuries such as Paracelsus, Maxwell, and Fludd, Mesmer believed that gravitational or magnetic forces in the body influenced health. Beginning first with magnets and later shifting to the "magnetic" forces within his own body, Mesmer believed that there is a "magnetic fluid" in all living matter and claimed he could cure others by affecting the balance of this fluid. In contrast to the occultists, who believed mental illness was caused by intrusion of outside agents or organic causes, Mesmer was convinced that the phenomenon of magnetic healing was not "backed up by an occult world view, but by a physical theory," and in this sense initiated a scientific investigation of the workings of the mind (Crabtree 1993:7).

The theory of animal magnetism would not itself have led to a study of the mind, however, were it not for the work of Marquis de Puységur, a disciple of Mesmer. Puységur discovered that magnetization could produce an altered state of consciousness—what he called "magnetic sleep." Puységur noted that this magnetic sleep differed from the normal state of consciousness. In the process of studying this nonconscious element of the mind, he began exploring the mental secrets of the magnetized subject as part of the healing process—what he considered an "alternate form of consciousness." Stressing the importance of the magnetist and of the relationship between therapist and subject, Puységur's technique foreshadowed the relationship in modern-day psychotherapy between therapist and client (Crabtree 1993:46–53).

Although by the end of the eighteenth century there was a large body of literature on the role of imagination in magnetic healing, as well as many scientific attempts to explain the growing phenomenon of magnetism, it was not until the work of James Braid and his conception of hypnotism that mesmerism took another turn. Braid, a Scottish doctor, noted that the phenomenon of mesmerism was largely physiological. Observing a magnetized subject, Braid observed that:

> ... the phenomena of mesmerism were to be accounted for on the principle of a derangement of the state of the cerebro-spinal centres, and of the circulatory, and respiratory, and muscular systems, induced... by a fixed stare, absolute repose of body, fixed attention, and suppressed respiration concomitant with that fixity of attention. That the whole depended on the physical and psychical condition of the patient, arising from the causes referred to, and not at all on the volition, or passes of the operator, throwing out a magnetic fluid, or exciting into activity some mystical universal fluid or medium (Braid 1899:101–2).

He called this state "nervous sleep," or hypnosis, and argued that the effects of this condition were therefore attributable entirely to physiology, and not to the special powers of the magnetist.

Based on his concept of hypnosis, Braid now developed what he considered a more legitimate form of therapy, or treatment, than the earlier form of magnetic healing. Describing hypnosis as a condition of mental "abstraction" or "concentration of attention, in which the powers of the mind are engrossed ... with a single idea or train of thought...," Braid now had discovered what he felt was a valuable therapeutic tool, based on a physiological process in which the mind can be used to affect the body:

> Since it cannot be doubted that the soul and the body can mutually act and react upon each other, it should follow, as a natural consequence, that if we can attain to any mode of intensifying the mental *power, we should thus realize, in a corresponding degree, greater control over physical action. Now this is precisely what my processes do—they create no new faculties; but they give us greater control over the natural functions than we possess during the ordinary waking condition and particularly in intensifying mental influence, or the power of the mind of the patient over his own physical functions... (Braid 1853:12).*

Hypnosis, then, makes it possible to extend the normal power of the mind. If a person's thoughts affect the body during ordinary waking conditions, this power must be even stronger when "the attention is so much more concentrated, and the imagination and faith, or expectant idea in the mind of the patient, are so much more intense than in the ordinary waking condition" (Braid 1853:3–4).

Hypnotism in France, particularly the work of Hippolyte Bernheim and the Nancy school, stressed that "hypnotism was a psychological state in its own right, one intimately connected with suggestion" (Crabree 1993:164). This focus on the central role of suggestion in hypnotism became widely accepted, and modern hypnosis, or hypnotherapy, is now commonly used in treating behavior disorders, addiction, anxiety, cardiovascular, gastrointestinal and other stress disorders, headaches, insomnia, pain, and emotional problems.

Psychoanalysis and Psychosomatic Medicine

One of the illnesses that received a great deal of attention as a result of the technique of hypnosis was hysteria—a particular set of inexplicable complaints that often occurred in women. Jean Martin Charcot, who systematized the study of hysteria, conceived the illness in purely physiological terms, leading to a broader acceptance of hysteria among doctors

(Crabtree 1993:166). At the same time, however, the study of hysteria was becoming increasingly a new discipline: the field of psychology, in which many of the same medically trained researchers were increasingly viewing hysteria as a psychological phenomenon that manifested in the form of physical symptoms.

Pierre Janet, for instance, believed that hysteria, like many psychological disturbances, was not adequately explained by physiology, but was connected with a dissociated element of the personality that was hidden from awareness. This hidden consciousness, he said, could produce actions for which the normal consciousness could not account. Defining an unconscious act as "an action having all the characteristics of a psychological act, save one: that it is always unknown by the person himself who executes it at the moment of its execution" (Janet 1889:225), Janet sought to unravel the structure and content of the different layers of consciousness.

Herbart, another early psychologist whose work foreshadowed that of Freud's, conceived of an unconscious "in terms of ideas of varying intensity—a notion which Freud later replaced by a conflict of affects..." (Jones 1953:372). Herbart also formulated a concept of repression and conceived of psychic forces that needed to be balanced, that were measurable and whose laws, through science, could be understood and clearly formulated.

The most important psychological theory relating to the study of unexplained physical problems emerged from the work of Sigmund Freud, who described, in his early studies with Breuer on hysteria, a mechanism for converting psychic conflict into physical symptoms:

> We must regard the process as though a sum of excitation impinging on the nervous system is transformed in chronic symptoms in so far as it has not been employed for external action in proportion to its amount. Now we are accustomed to find in hysteria that a considerable part of this 'sum of excitation' of the trauma is transformed into purely somatic symptoms. It is this characteristic of hysteria which has so long stood in the way of its being recognized as a psychical disorder (Breuer et al. 1974:146).

This "transformation of psychical excitation into chronic somatic symptoms" Freud called "conversion." This "intentional repression is also the basis for the conversion.... The sum of excitation, being cut off from psychical association, finds its way all the more easily along the wrong path to a somatic innervation" (146). In other words, repressed mental energy manifests in the form of physical symptoms.

Extending his work on the psychic roots of physical symptoms, Freud developed the field of psychoanalysis—the study of the unconscious mind. The method of psychoanalysis is based primarily on the "talking cure"— the technique of talking about apparently insignificant phenomena and, through the process of free association, bringing out feelings and problems in order to expose repressed memories which hold the key to neurotic symptoms.

Extending the insights of psychoanalysis to include stress-related illness, Franz Alexander observed that many real illnesses are in fact based on emotional distress—what he called "vegetative neurosis." The role of emotions in illness had long been recognized by doctors and healers. But Alexander insisted that the role of emotions in causing illness, in light of psychoanalytic insights, was now capable of being studied scientifically, and as such should be considered a legitimate branch of medicine, one in which a "detailed knowledge of the relationship between emotional life and body processes extends the function of the physician" (Alexander 1950:48). In contrast to the psychosomatic symptoms of hysteria, vegetative neurosis is in fact a stress disease, but one in which "emotional factors are of causal significance" (43). Contrasting the two, Alexander writes,

> A conversion symptom is a symbolic expression of an
> emotionally charged psychological content: it is an attempt to
> discharge the emotional tension.... A vegetative neurosis is not
> an attempt to express an emotion but is the physiological
> response of the vegetative organs to constant or to periodically
> returning emotional states (42).

In thus identifying the role of emotional states in such stress-related conditions as heart and respiratory disease and gastrointestinal disorders, Alexander was one of the pioneers of a new field in the study of stress—the study of psychosomatic medicine.

A popular recent example of a psychosomatic theory of stress is John Sarno's theory of back pain. Challenging the view that structural abnormalities cause back pain, Sarno observes that in fact "common emotional situations" bring about a "physiologic alteration in certain muscles, nerves, tendons and ligaments which is called the Tension Myositis Syndrome (TMS)" (Sarno 1991:3). According to Sarno, back pain is a recognizable physiologic syndrome, but it is a syndrome caused by "repressed emotions" and serves "to prevent them from becoming conscious" (48). The brain then chooses "from among a large repertoire of painful and non-painful disorders when it needs to defend against painful or undesirable feelings" (146). Focusing as it does on defenses against feelings, Sarno's view is a variation of Alexander's psychosomatic theory, the difference being in his elaboration on the role of emotions on stress and physiological states in the body.

Behaviorism

It is well known that responses to stressful stimuli can evoke a condition which, if persistent and unrelieved, can eventually lead to illness. When once one considers, though, that many stimuli are not in and of themselves harmful, then the response to a stimulus must (at least in many cases) be viewed as learned. The concept of learned behavior, emerging from the biological and evolutionary study of behavior, was first advanced as a behavioral concept by E. Thorndike: "Any act which in a given situation produces satisfaction becomes associated with that situation, so that when the situation recurs the act is more likely than before to recur also" (Thorndike 1905:203). Ivan Pavlov concretized this concept in his experiments on digestion in dogs. Noting that dogs began salivating when they heard food coming, he concluded that the dog must have been "conditioned to expect food before it actually arrived" (Pavlov 1927). This study of "conditioned reflexes" led to the concept of "reinforcement," or stamping in of conditioned responses over repeated experiences.

These observations give credence to the view that stress is a maladaptive, learned response. If a particular stimulus is repeatedly accompanied by a painful experience such as a shock, we will become sensitized to that stimulus; even when the experience ceases to be painful, we will respond to it with the same anxiety and avoidance as we did to the original event. In some cases, responses to stress can be weakened by learning to relax and then being progressively exposed to the "anxiety-provoking stimulus" under controlled conditions—a process called "systematic desensitization" (Wolpe 1958). Conditioning theory has also demonstrated that when an animal has been given low levels of stimulation during infancy and development, it responds to a wider range of stressors, and with more "severely damaging consequences" (Levine 1960). In contrast, when the painful stimulus is accompanied by a warning signal and accompanied by positive feedback, then stress levels return to virtually the same level as the groups that received no shocks at all (Levine 1971).

This behavioral view contrasts sharply with the psychoanalytic concept of neurosis. Because "neurotic behavior demonstrably originates in learning, it is only to be expected that its elimination will be a matter of unlearning" (Wolpe 1958:ix); a true psychotherapy could therefore dispense with the notion of inner mental processes and could proceed on the basis of learning theory alone. Culminating with Skinner, the behaviorists asserted that behaviorism "can safely throw out a real challenge to the subjective psychologists—show us that you have a possible method, indeed that you have a legitimate subject-matter" (Watson 1925:17). In its ultimate form, behaviorism thus rejected psychology as the study of the mind and of consciousness, and settled the mind-body question by asserting that since all learning can be explained on the basis of conditioning alone, neither mind nor consciousness in fact exist.

Body-Oriented Psychotherapy

By its very nature, the field of psychology, beginning with the study of hypnotism, was focused on establishing the reality of an undetected mental life—a trend that, even with the development of physiology, has continued for many decades. In the latter half of the twentieth century, however, a number of psychologists attempted to establish the body as the focal point of psychological insight. The link between physiology and psychology can be traced at least as far back as the classical doctrine in Greek medicine of four humors—blood, phlegm, yellow bile, and black bile—which became associated with the four temperaments—sanguine, phlegmatic, choleric, and melancholic—found in later Greek literature (Philips 1973:52). Also of note is the work of W. H. Sheldon, who described three classifications of human physiques, or "somatotypes" (endomorph, ectomorph, and mesomorph), each of which, perhaps harking back to the ancient Greek concept of body humors, he linked to temperamental qualities (Sheldon 1940, 1942).

Another psychologist whose work foreshadows the body-oriented psychotherapies of the twentieth century is Paul Schilder, who coined the term "body image" to denote how the "image of body is constructed" (Schilder 1950:286). Wanting to "consider the body as an entity and as a unit" (283), he also notes that "many types of muscular tone influence the postural model of the body" (78). Schilder also says that "it is clear that every emotion expresses itself in the postural model of the body, and that every expressive attitude is connected with characteristic changes in the postural model of the body" (209).

The body as the focal point of psychology came to fruition in the work of Wilhelm Reich, a psychoanalyst trained by Freud. Exploring the basis of resistance in his patients, Reich observed that "a basic conflict which a person experienced at a certain stage of life left its trace in his character in the form of a defensive rigidity of attitude, behavior and expression" (Boadella 1975:43); "...the patient's character...becomes the resistance against the uncovering of the unconscious" (Reich 1972:154). Later, Reich took this theory a step further by claiming that "sexual life energy can be bound by chronic muscular tensions" (Reich 1961:242), and his treatment gradually directed "more and more attention to the state of tension in the body musculature" (Boadella 1975:120), culminating in his "vegetative" technique of working on the musculature in order to release pent-up emotions and resolve psychic conflict.

Body armoring, as Reich conceived it, is not to be confused with the concept of conversion in traditional psychoanalytic theory. In conversion, psychic conflict is forced into somatic channels, so that a mental conflict manifests in the form of a symptom that is not "real," but a secondary problem that merely hints at an underlying conflict. Muscular armoring, in contrast, is a series of constrictions whose direct function is to limit movement and feeling (Boadella 1975:121).

Alexander Lowen further popularized Reich's work by developing a system called Bioenergetics for mobilizing the energies in individuals whose forms of expression have become in some way blocked or disturbed. Unlike psychotherapies that use primarily verbal techniques for exploring neurotic problems, bioenergetic therapy is concerned with the total expressive behavior of a person, manifested in bodily movements and the fundamental rhythmic processes of the body, especially breathing. His approach, as with a number of others that have since developed, focuses more "on the release of muscular tension than on giving in to sexual feelings" (Lowen 1976:39). The system utilizes a combination of deep breathing exercises, talk therapy, massage, and muscular exercises to release repressed emotions and associated chronic muscular tensions and armoring.

Stress, Relaxation, and Behavioral Medicine

a. Evolutionary Theory

It is well known that when faced with danger an animal has two choices —to run or to fight—and that accompanying these responses are autonomic physiological changes that prepare the animal for heightened activity. The term "fight or flight response" was first coined by Walter Cannon, who observed that there is an automatic response accompanying fear and rage—namely, increased discharge of adrenalin and sugar, increased heart rate, and improved muscle tone—and that the main purpose of this response is to enable an animal to survive in the face of unforeseen dangers (Cannon 1939,1967).

Due to the development of such introspective psychologies as psychoanalysis, emotions are now often viewed as subjective or psychic states. But emotion, as Cannon conceived it, evolved in an evolutionary context, and within the context of the struggle for survival; and in fact the fight-flight concept has its origins in evolutionary theory. In Darwin, for instance, "certain complex actions are of direct or indirect service under certain states of the mind," and are therefore serviceable in achieving actual ends, or at least once were (Darwin 1965:28). As Spencer wrote, "Fear, when strong, expresses itself in cries, in efforts to hide or escape, in palpitations and tremblings; and these are just the manifestations that would accompany an actual experience of the evil feared" (Spencer 1899:482). The states of fear and rage, therefore, have a direct function in the context of survival, and this gives rise to the concept of fight or flight. And as McDougall suggested, an association has become established between particular emotions and particular instinctive reactions; thus the emotion of fear is associated with the instinct for flight, and the emotion of anger or rage with the instinct for fighting or attack. A connection therefore exists between "flight instinct" and "fear emotion," and the "pugnacity instinct" and "anger emotion" (McDougall 1908:49–50).

b. Medical Research

Although early evolutionary biologists observed the physiological reactions associated with fighting enemies and fleeing from predators, it was Cannon who first described the actual physiological changes that accompanied these responses, and in so doing gave rise to the concept of a physiology of stress. He argued that since fear and anger in wildlife are likely to be followed by vigorous activity—namely, running or fighting—the physiological response that accompanies these states is of service to the animal in the struggle for survival. "The conclusion seems justified, therefore, that the increased blood sugar attendant on the major emotions and pain would be of direct benefit to the organism in the strenuous muscular efforts involved in flight or conflict or struggle to be free" (Cannon 1939:202–3). Like other regulatory mechanisms in the body, this response enables the body to maintain itself internally and in relation to the environment. Studying the bodily mechanisms for adjustment to the environment, Cannon thus formulated the idea of *homeostasis,* which he describes as the "coordinated physiological processes which maintain most of the steady states in the organism" (Cannon 1967:24); the "fight or flight response" was one such mechanism.

When viewed as a homeostatic mechanism, the fight-flight response operates as a normal regulatory function. Hans Selye, however, observed that the stress response can often be deleterious. In contrast to specific disease that manifests in relation to particular germ invaders or other identifiable causes, the body, Selye claimed, has a general nonspecific reaction pattern, called the "general adaptation syndrome," or "stress syndrome," that it uses to meet various forms of damage. Identifying this response as "the common denominator of all adaptive reactions in the body," Selye observed that these symptoms had been observed but never fully understood or medically studied; by studying these reactions as a general syndrome, he identified specific characteristics of this adaptive response, such as adrenal stimulation, regulation of blood pressure, and metabolic changes. Selye thus identified various ailments such as arthritis, heart disease, and digestive and metabolic disorders as diseases of maladaptation, and assigned "the body's own defensive adaptive reactions," not the presence of specific illness, as the cause. Selye thus established the modern concept of stress as a maladaptive condition not caused by disease in the form of outside germ invaders, but by our own harmful adaptive response to stress (Selye 1956).

c. Stress-Reduction Techniques

Based on the concept of stress, many techniques have been developed for muscle relaxation and control. Biofeedback, for instance, is "the process or technique for learning voluntary control over automatically regulated body functions," by "'feeding back' physiological information to the individual generating the information" (Brown 1977:3). Perhaps the earliest use of biofeedback training was made centuries ago by yogis learning to regulate their basal metabolism. This phenomenon was studied in the early twentieth century by Johannes H. Schultz, who developed a form of relaxation based on autohypnosis and visualization called Autogenic Training. By observing how "the psychophysiologic mechanisms" could be "mobilized by autosuggestions" (Schultz et al. 1959), Schultz developed a method for gaining self-control over specific organs, physiological states, and brain function.

In the 1920s, Edmund Jacobsen observed electrical activity in muscles and developed a method for training people to reduce this tension. In 1934, Olive Smith described the conscious control of individual motor unit potentials, followed by D. B. Lindsley, who confirmed his findings and showed that electrical activity in muscles could be completely eliminated. In 1962, John Basmajian, who popularized the technique of biofeedback, reported that if the electrical activity in the motor units of particular muscles is displayed either visually or with audio feedback by using electromyography (EMG), it is possible very quickly to learn to control the activity in these muscles (Basmajian 1962:62). Interestingly, Basmajian wrote, "no one who can control single-motor-unit firing can describe how it is done…" (Green et al.:31–2); the fact remains, however, that in the many cases where it has been successful, "single cells were being controlled by volition" (32). EMG biofeedback thus provides a remarkable demonstration of the physiological concreteness of thought processes, as well as the role of awareness and volition in learning to control muscle tension.

Currently "the most useful of all the biofeedback techniques," EMG biofeedback has been reported to be effective in treating a wide range of disorders such as anxiety, phobias, tension headaches, temporomandibular joint syndrome (TMJ), insomnia, essential hypertension, and digestive problems (Brown 1977:52–55). Biofeedback has also been used to control brain waves (first observed in the nineteenth century and later described by Hans Berger as *alpha, beta, delta* and *theta* waves) as well as heart rate, blood pressure, and other autonomic functions (Brown 1977; Green et al. 1977; Caton 1875; Kamiya 1968, 1969).

Another method for relieving stress is Edmund Jacobsen's technique of "progressive relaxation." Based on tightening specific muscles and then learning to sense kinesthetically the tension in the muscle, the method sought to progressively and systematically relax muscles throughout the body. Defining relaxation as the "opposite physiologically to excitation of muscles" (Jacobsen 1962:*ix*), Jacobsen applied his technique to a wide variety of symptoms such as fear, anxiety, hypertension, ulcers, and nervous disorders. Because activity requires muscle tension, he taught the individual to relax during everyday activities by learning to relax muscles not directly involved in the activity—a process he termed "differential relaxation" (124–129).

Jacobsen also believed muscular tension was the cause of nervous and mental disorders. Observing electrical impulses present in muscles during contraction, he believed that tension was the equivalent of overactive nerves (85). Since tension in muscles increases susceptibility to reaction, the "cause" of stress or various nervous disorders is not the external stimulus, but the tension itself. He thus challenged the view that mental states or outside circumstances cause tension (as expressed in the popular conception that worry causes tension, or the psychoanalytic view that subjective conflict manifests in bodily form) and instead contended that "nervous disturbance equals mental disturbance" *(ix)*. In studying anxiety, Jacobsen also observed that ideas correspond to action with "faint and abbreviated muscular acts" (168); muscular tension, therefore, "is a *sine quo non* of imagery, attention and thought-process" (Jacobsen 1938:186). By relaxing muscles, the thinking associated with the muscular activity stops, and so do mental problems: "...[an] emotional state fails to exist in the presence of complete relaxation of the peripheral parts involved" (Jacobsen 1938:218).

Another technique for reducing stress was developed by Herbert Benson. Benson noted that hypertension is influenced not simply by diet and weight but by situations requiring behavioral readjustment, which in turn invoke the fight-flight response. However, Benson argued, the hyperactivity of the sympathetic nervous system associated with fight-or-flight can be countered by relaxation techniques, such as the mantra meditation of transcendental meditation (TM), which quiet the sympathetic nervous system (Benson 1975:73). Because the restful state associated with lowered sympathetic activity is the "opposite" of the heightened fight-flight activity, Benson concludes that the regular use of meditation— what he termed the "relaxation response"—will offset the harmful effects of the stress response (94–96).

Other methods for reducing stress focus on behavior and belief systems. Friedman and Rosenman, for instance, observed that a consistent pattern of behavior (which they called the Type A personality) was closely associated with coronary heart disease. They recommended a process of consciously altering attitudes and belief systems (Friedman et al. 1974). Simonton and Simonton have observed that cancers can be reduced by employing relaxation and imagery, suggesting that "since psychologic stress has been shown to depress immune activity, it seems logical to postulate that stress reduction and the mobilization of positive psychological attitudes may be one means of restoring the body's ability to overcome invasive viruses and destroy mutant cells" (Pelletier 1982:252).

Holistic Medicine

Although it has enjoyed a recent popularity, holistic medicine has been practiced in various forms for centuries. Hippocrates, often called the "father of Western medicine," expressed a holistic view when he recognized the human body's ability to heal itself without the intervention of a doctor *(vis medicatrix naturae)*. He also believed that the main role of the doctor was to avoid treatment that might interfere with this process, and above all to do no harm *(primum non nocere)*. Various shamanic practices also view physical illness as an expression of spiritual or moral conflict, and thus treat illness "holistically." In its modern form,

> ... *holistic medicine recognizes the inextricable interaction between the person and his psychosocial environment. Mind and body function as an integrated unit, and health exists when they are in harmony, while illness results when stress and conflict disrupt this process. These approaches are essentially humanistic and reestablish an emphasis upon the patient rather than upon medical technology. Modern medicine has tended to view man as a machine with interchangeable parts, and has developed sophisticated procedures for repairing, removing, or artificially constructing these parts. These are significant achievements, but in the process the healing professions have lost sight of man as a dynamic, integrated, and complex system with a marked capacity for self-healing (Pelletier 1982:11–12).*

Holistic medicine employs a number of concepts and practices. The first is the concept of balance. Since health is affected by many factors, treatment must include attention to, and the balancing of, many internal forces, including personality, stress and hereditary factors, diet, exercise, and life situations. This balance is achieved by borrowing from traditional naturalistic practices such as Ayurvedic medicine, traditional Chinese medicine, and homeopathy, all of which are based on a concept of self-regulation, balance, and the body's inherent ability to adjust itself.

A second essential feature of holistic medicine is the employment of various techniques to consciously regulate excessive stress such as meditation, yoga, relaxation, biofeedback, autogenic training, and visualization, all of which produce a "sustained period of diminished sympathetic activity with an attendant increase in parasympathetic activity" and "relaxation of skeletal muscles, decreased blood pressure and respiration rate" (Pelletier 1982:119).

A third factor is recognition of the role of mental attitude and consciousness in healing. Doctors and healers in various cultures have long recognized the influence of mental attitude and emotions on health. Hippocrates, for instance, felt that imagery and physical processes were intimately linked. Doctors have also recognized for centuries that many digestive diseases are related to emotional distress and that, even in purely physical illnesses, the role of positive thinking, faith in God, or belief in the doctor can have a direct impact on recovery. Holistic medicine consciously employs the power of thought to reduce stress and to strengthen the body's immune function. Norman Cousins, for instance, gives a personal account of his illness and of the power of laughter and his will to live which, he said, "is not a theoretical abstraction, but a physiologic reality with therapeutic characteristics" (Cousins 1980:44). Another more metaphysical view of the role of consciousness in healing is Deepak Chopra's anti-mechanistic view of health and the human body. Combining modern scientific research with ancient Ayurvedic concepts, Chopra speaks of the "quantum mechanical body"—the "invisible software that shapes, controls, and creates the physical self" (Chopra 1990:107). Borrowing from scientific studies that demonstrate the link between thought process and physiology, Chopra argues that because consciousness determines how our body functions, the "real medicine our bodies need is medicine for our awareness" (109). "If you look closely at the your own life," Chopra writes, "you will realize that you are sending signals to your body that repeat the same old beliefs, the same old fears and wishes, the same old habits of yesterday and the day before" (310).

By utilizing our own conscious awareness, Chopra argues, we can alter our entire health with the "inner intelligence that knows how to build your heart, kidneys, skin, enzymes, hormones, DNA, and everything else. This intelligence is literally infinite, and all of it is under our control" (311). According to Chopra, then, health is a reflection of consciousness; by altering our belief systems, we can ultimately reverse illness.

Yoga, Meditation, and Oriental Medicine

Oriental medicine, which has been practiced in many forms for several thousand years, is based on philosophical principles which, in a very general sense, recognize the unity of mind and body as well as the influence of personality, emotion, and thought on physical health. These traditional forms are inextricably linked with philosophical and religious concepts, as well as spiritual practices, which I will briefly summarize.

a. Ayurvedic Medicine

Meaning "knowledge for longevity," Ayurvedic medicine is a system of medical and spiritual practices based on an ancient tradition and extensive literature. According to Ayurveda, the human organism is governed by three humors (*vata, pitta,* and *kapha*), analogous to the four Greek humors, which must be in balance in order to maintain health, but which often become imbalanced due to improper diet, environment, and other factors. By assigning "a particular set of characteristics to each person according to his or her discomfort and constitutional makeup," the practitioner identifies imbalances in these three humors and "applies various natural agents in order to restore equilibrium" (Das et al. 1978:53).

Ayurvedic techniques include herbal medicines, massage, ointments, diet and purification, meditation, and Hatha yoga. Ayurvedic medicine also takes into account the role of conduct, emotions, and behavior, and in this sense is more than a therapy; it is a "science and art of appropriate living" (Das et al. 1978:53).

b. Yoga, Meditation, and Healing Techniques

Yoga, which is popularly known in the West as a system of physical exercises, in fact embraces a huge *corpus* of teaching and practice spanning many centuries. Spiritual insight, not physical exercise, is the basis for yoga:

> *Meditation is at the very heart of yoga. Sitting quietly, and just thinking about a situation, a person, a project or a problem is the simplest form of meditation.... From this simple form of meditation, which is highly beneficial from its effect of both stimulating and relaxing at the same time, other forms have developed (Worthington 1982:100).*

The most popular yoga practice among Westerners is Hatha yoga, which comprises physical postures and exercises taught for improved health and well-being. The various postures of Hatha yoga were originally associated with the breath, and they were "considered entirely secondary and subservient to the main practice, which was sitting for meditation with the object of eventually achieving *samadhi* (enlightenment)" (Worthington 1982:128). In the Tantric period, however, "more active exercises began to be employed," largely to improve the "general health of yoga practitioners," and came to refer to "the whole range of yoga physical exercises" (128).

In early writings on yoga, various practitioners describe an energy "rising from the base of the spine" and having a "cleansing and vitalizing effect on the whole system" (100). This energy was later described in terms of "chakras," or energy centers, organized at various points along the spine, and corresponding to various emotions and personality traits. In Laya yoga, meditative techniques are used to "cleanse and activate this energy system," and have since been practiced in order "to activate, sedate or generally heal the body and mind" (101). A number of modern healing techniques are aimed at influencing the chakras and kundalini energy arising from the base of the spine through sound, crystals, touch, and other methods. Reiki and touch therapy are examples of contemporary healing techniques that are related to ancient yoga practices, and which seek to activate and balance the energy systems. Other meditation techniques focus on awakening the vital center of the abdomen, known as *hara* to the Japanese, as the basis for health and spiritual insight.

Breath control also plays a large part in yoga. Yogic philosophy maintains that "the entire nervous system is nourished and toned up" when breathing takes place correctly (Kamananda 1976:143). By practicing various *pranayamas,* or breathing exercises, the subject establishes correct breathing, deepens concentration and the ability to meditate, and brings about a relaxed and vitalized condition. Meditation is also complemented by *asanas,* or meditative postures, which complement mental discipline.

Mantra yoga, or Transcendental Meditation (mentioned earlier in the work of Benson on stress), is a meditation technique that is also widely used as a means of relaxation. The practitioner is given a "mantra," a word or phrase in Sanskrit, and meditates by focusing on the mantra. In doing this, "the metabolic rate falls below the level of sleep. The heartbeat slows down, but at the same time the flow of oxygen increases, while brainwave patterns show a simultaneous effect of deep relaxation with high alertness" (Kamananda 1976:144).

c. Chinese Medicine

Best known for the practice of acupuncture, Chinese medicine in fact incorporates a large array of techniques that are, in turn, based on broad philosophical principles. At the heart of Chinese medicine is the concept of energy, or *chi,* which ebbs and flows in all of nature in the form of *yin* and *yang.* The human being, according to Taoist philosophy, is endowed with "three treasures": body, energy, and spirit. When the individual lives in balance and harmony both with nature and internally, then the *chi,* which flows in each person and is the vital source for all basic organ functions, is in balance, and the "three treasures" are guarded. When, however, the balance of *chi* is disturbed, then the three treasures are in danger, and degeneration and disease can result (Reid 1994).

Chinese medicine recognizes a number of factors in the maintenance of balanced *chi.* External influences such as weather and environment, as well as diet, can directly influence the balance of *yin* and *yang.* Internal influences such as "excessive" emotions, lack of moderation in habits of living, and overindulgence in food, as well as spiritual conflict, can also cause imbalances in the *chi.*

Chinese medicine employs various techniques, such as herbs and massage, for restoring the balance of *chi.* Acupuncture, through the use of needles, directly influences the flow of *chi* along meridians in the body, and restores the balance of *yin* and *yang*. Energy can be balanced and restored also through attention to one's behavior and through specific exercises and meditation. Qi Gong, or "energy work," is a system of exercises for regulating and correcting imbalances in *yin* and *yang*. Tai Chi, a series of movements related to the martial arts, is also widely practiced in China as a way of maintaining health and balancing energy. Finally, meditation is also used as a means of restoring the balance of *chi* as well as achieving spiritual maturity and insight, which in Taoist and Chinese philosophy is considered the ultimate means of ensuring longevity and health (Reid 1994:279–80).

Developmental Movement

Many techniques in the field of dance and movement include elements aimed at relaxation and increased control. The study of developmental movement, however, has a particular bearing on the study of mind and body. If *homo sapiens* and other species evolved from a common form of life, then it follows that the individual reflects in its singular development the passage through prior stages of evolutionary growth ("ontogeny recapitulates phylogeny," to use the famous phrase coined by Chambers). In the first few months of life, for instance, an infant exhibits reflex patterns of movement in the limbs which reflect those of amphibians and reptiles. Recognizing that these primitive reflexes are intact in patients who have damage to the higher cortex, Bobath, Fay, and others developed techniques, termed "neuro-developmental therapy," for restoring movement in children afflicted with cerebral palsy. By uncovering and employing basic patterns of movements, the "origin and evolution of human movement from the primitive past" (Fay 1955:644) can thus be utilized in "retraining and recoordinating the muscle groups in cases of cerebral palsy" (Fay 1948:330).

Observing that reading problems and other neurologic difficulties in children often seemed to reflect the inadequate passage through developmental stages of movement, Glenn Doman and Carl Delacato argue that "when we have seen a child who did not go through each of the major stages in the order in which they are listed, however briefly they may have remained in a stage, we have seen a child who later on gave evidence of having a major or a minor neurological problem" (Doman 1974:47). Inadequate or incomplete neurological organization," then, held the key to neurologic development:

> We had assumed that functions and performance were the result of brain development. Was it possible that brain development was the result of functions and performance? For instance, we had assumed that a healthy brain made it possible to walk, but could it be that the process of going through the stages toward walking is what created the complete and intact brain? (Delacato 1971:50).

Based on these observations, Doman and Delacato developed a technique, called "patterning," that helped a child to recover movement patterns that had been missed or inadequately developed, and in this way to improve "neurological organization."

Following the work of Bobath, Fay, Doman, and Delacato, a number of people have developed systems of awareness to be used in normal adults, to help reorganize the nervous system through the use of developmental movement. Raymond Dart, for instance, believed that malposture and the lack of poise in human adults "is the result of inadequately exploiting, of short-circuiting, or of actually eliminating the ancestral phases of posture...during ontogeny" (Dart 1996:26). Based on these observations, he recommends various postures and developmental movements, corresponding to the phases of evolving into the upright posture, which lead to improved "equilibration of the body" (28).

Bonnie Bainbridge Cohen, a dancer and occupational therapist, borrowed from principles of developmental movement to develop an awareness system called "Body-Mind Centering." Observing the various systems in the body from the point of view of movement and expression, Bainbridge Cohen helps people develop greater awareness and "mind-body integration." Many "adults are limited in how many of the basic perceptual-motor patterns (including the developmental movement patterns) they can do" (Bainbridge Cohen 1993:99). There are "developmental underlies to any problem...." (99); "... the next time you see a knee

problem," Bainbridge Cohen writes, "look for the developmental process underneath it" (104). By reorganizing patterns of movement, the brain
is similarly reorganized. As Cohen says, "I think that all mind pattern-
ings are expressed in movement, through the body. And that all physically moving patterns have a mind. That's what I work with" (103).

Various dance techniques, borrowing from the study of movement and
development, provide approaches to mind and body worth mentioning
because of their broadly educational intent. Labananalysis, the movement
notation system developed by Rudolph Laban, "provides a means of
perceiving and a vocabulary for describing movement—quantitatively
and qualitatively—that is applicable to any body movement research…"
(Bartenieff 1980:*viii*). Today his technique is applied not only to the dance,
but as a form of movement education applicable to general improvement of functional activity. Irmgard Bartenieff, a dancer and physical
therapist who, like Bainbridge Cohen, also drew upon her experiences
in rehabilitation, developed the Bartenieff Fundamentals—a system of
movements that "provide exercises for the experience of the body in
motion with an awareness of how and why it is moving" (20).

Body Awareness Techniques

In contrast to techniques that reduce stress directly by means of therapeutic treatment, there are a number of methods designed to improve
movement patterns and bodily functioning through awareness. Mabel
Todd developed an unconventional approach to movement education that
widened the scope of most exercise, posture, and movement programs.
Based "upon the concurrent study of physics, mechanics, anatomy and
physiology," Todd's approach seeks to improve posture, balance, and muscular function by correctly conceiving of the anatomical and functional
structures of the body. Although her work includes detailed descriptions
of breathing, physiology, proprioception, and mechanical analysis of balance and forces in the body, her approach centers largely on the skeletal
system. "Knowledge of the natural forces in its dynamic balances" is
"the way to conservation and a more efficient use of human energy" (Todd
1937:295). "Bodily balance in accord with the principles of mechanics,"
she writes, "is a poignant means for conservation of nervous energy" (*xiv*).

Correct conceptual knowledge of anatomical function, then, becomes the basis for efficient movement and increased awareness and control.

The Feldenkrais method, developed by Moshe Feldenkrais, employs simple movements to bring about more efficient paths of mobility and to integrate sensory and motor functions through kinesthetic awareness. It also employs subtle manipulation on a one-to-one level to bring about changes in coordination and awareness. Drawing from his own background in martial arts and from physiological knowledge of the nervous system, particularly as it applies to movement, Feldenkrais argued that a more complete approach to personality could be developed by dropping "the arbitrary assumption that mental processes alone are sufficient to give a full account of the personality, and by taking somatic processes into account" (Feldenkrais 1949:35). Focusing on behavior as a function of the developing nervous system, Feldenkrais argued that the key to "personality readjustment" is "muscular and postural re-education" that removes "emotional and bodily blocks to maturity and spontaneity based on function" (163). The main problem, Feldenkrais argued, is emotional upheavals in early life that force the child to adopt attitudes of flexor contraction and extensor inhibition; psychiatric methods alone will not change this underlying "muscular and attitudinal" pattern. By performing various movements that redistribute muscle tone and promote new patterns of movement and action, the "muscular anxiety pattern is broken up by a proper distribution of habitual tone between flexors and antigravity muscles" (156). By thus stimulating new movement patterns, the brain is similarly stimulated, increasing mental flexibility, intelligence and, ultimately, maturity.

Gerda Alexander developed a technique of sensory and bodily awareness, called Eutony, that addressed the whole person. Influenced by the work of Jacques Dalcroze, founder of the technique of music education based on rhythm and movement, Alexander expanded these concepts into a general method for developing bodily and sensory awareness and improved sensory and emotional contact with the environment and other people. Her view was that "the general involuntary tonus regulation and the autonomic balance can be consciously influenced" through awareness, and that this leads to experiencing the "unity of the total person"

(Alexander 1985:20). Such a process, Alexander argued, enabled the individual to overcome emotional fixations, to increase expressiveness, and to remove the cause of various chronic physical problems. Such a process, she claimed, impacted on chronic ailments as well as emotional fixations, which could be eliminated through a process of developing a more accurate body image and regaining sensory and emotional contact.

Elsa Gindler and Charlotte Selver developed a system called Sensory Awareness. Recovering from a bout with tuberculosis that had adversely affected her health, Gindler "practiced the sensitive attention to breathing, posture, and movement that formed the basis of her later work" (Murphy 1993:405). Linking the calm condition achieved in this state with changes in emotion, she came to believe that "calm (or trust) in the physical field is equivalent to trust in the psychic field" (405). The technique is based on focused kinesthetic awareness, which she felt facilitated functioning: "Awareness of kinesthetic feedback from our neural system predisposes the muscular system to adjust itself to more efficient functioning.... [Then] the changed motor patterns cycle back and give new sensory impressions, which again readjust the muscular coordination, and so on..." (406). In the United States, Gindler's work was spread by Charlotte Selver. The method, which Fritz Perls later incorporated into his Gestalt therapy, is not structured, but is based on empirical, or exploratory, observation of oneself.

Massage and Bodywork Techniques

In recent years, massage and bodywork techniques have been promoted not only as part of a holistic health regimen but as a means of addressing the unity of mind and body by increasing sensorimotor awareness and reducing stress. Bodywork techniques have also been developed as a "somatic" approach to emotional work and utilized in conjunction with psychotherapeutic techniques.

Massage has been practiced in India, China, Greece, and throughout the world for many centuries. One of the earliest works on massage is *The Yellow Emperor's Classic of Internal Medicine,* dating to 1,000 B.C., which advocates the use of massage in treatment of various illnesses. Although widely used in ancient times in the treatment of various disorders, Hippocrates was one of the first to discuss the use of massage and its contra-indications (Kamenetz 1980:4–8). Massage and bodywork practices comprise a vast array of techniques and are used today to promote general relaxation, improve circulation and mobilize joints, relieve stress and muscle tension, and to enhance a general sense of well-being in the client.

A number of bodywork techniques focus on deep tissue manipulation. A particularly influential form of bodywork is Structural Integration, or Rolfing, developed by Ida Rolf. Rolf defines her technique as a

> ... ten-hour cycle of deep manual intervention in the elastic soft tissue structure (myofascia) of the body. The goal of this treatment is balance of the body in the gravity field; the principle of the treatment is, in brief, that if tissue is restrained, and balanced movement demanded at a nearby joint, tissue and joint will relocate in a more appropriate equilibrium (Rolf 1977:11).

Believing that the structure of the body holds the key to many emotional and physical imbalances, Rolf argued that "emotional response is behavior, is function. All behavior is expressed through the musculoskeletal system. All function is an expression of structure and form and correlates directly with material structure" (17). Speaking of the relation of mind and body, Rolf writes:

> The premise of modern psychotherapy is that man's outer circumstances are the projection of his inner, often hidden, self. This premise may be looked at from a different angle: a man's emotional state may be seen as the projection of his structural imbalances.... A man who undergoes integration of his corporeal structure experiences the basic link that exists between structure and emotion (17–18).

In other words, "... emotion reflects physical material balance or imbalance" (280). Since the work of Rolf, a number of variants to Rolfing have evolved which supplement bodywork techniques with movement and awareness education, as well as psychological work incident to the release of unconscious holding patterns in the body (Hellerwork and

Aston Patterning are two such examples) (Heller et al. 1991; Aston 1991, 1993).

Trager is a gentle, nonmanipulative form of bodywork that uses touch to facilitate awareness and to release tension arising from fixed patterns of emotional and physical holding. Its concern is

"... not with moving particular muscles or joints per se, *but with using motion in muscles and joints to produce particular sensory feelings—positive, pleasurable feelings which enter the central nervous system and begin to trigger tissue changes by means of the many sensory-motor feedback loops between the mind and the muscles" (Juhan 1987a:1).*

Observing that touch had the power of accessing the person's unconscious and bringing about pleasurable feelings of healing and release, Trager designed his work as a means of reaching the mental or unconscious aspects of the physical holding. Quoting Trager, Juhan writes, "The pattern of stiffness and of aging exists more in the unconscious than in the tissues" (Juhan 1987a:6). "I am convinced," Trager says,

... that for every physical non-yielding condition there is a psychic counterpart in the unconscious mind corresponding exactly to the degree of the physical manifestation.... These patterns often develop in response to adverse circumstances such as accidents, surgery, illness, poor posture, emotional trauma, stresses of daily living, or poor movement habits. The purpose of my work is to break up these sensory and mental patterns which inhibit free movement and cause pain and disruption of normal function (Juhan 1992:3).

In this sense, Juhan asserts, the Trager approach is a "subtle and intuitive approach to the elusive and complex problem of the physiological manifestation of psychological distress" (Juhan 1987a:7).

A number of Oriental or meridian-based bodywork techniques focus not on the concept of muscle armoring but on energy flow. Based on the concept of *chi,* Shiatsu employs deep pressure along the acupuncture meridians to remove blockage and restore normal flow of energy.

Acupressure, which is like acupuncture but does not involve the use of needles to stimulate energy points along the meridians, employs pressure from the fingers and hands for the same purpose. In stimulating energy points in this way, acupressure aims to remove the energy blocks that produce health problems (Burton Goldberg Group 1993).

Polarity therapy, developed by Dr. Randolph Stone, is another bodywork technique based on a concept of energy similar to the Oriental concept of *chi*. Believing that imbalances in life energy and disease result from armoring and repressed emotion, wrong diet, and stress, Stone's method seeks to balance this energy through an integration of Eastern and Western techniques, including manipulation of pressure points and joints, massage, breathwork, hydrotherapy, reflexology, stretching and other exercises, and the holding of energy points on the body to release blockages and restore the natural flow of energy (Binik 1978:53).

Performance Techniques and Rehearsal Imagery

It is well known among athletes that clear mental imaging of movements often facilitates the body's ability to carry out desired actions. Many athletes spend time before a match in a relaxed state, imagining exactly how they will execute a particular performance. Jack Nicklaus reported that he "never hit a shot, not even in practice, without having a very sharp, in-focus picture of it in my head" (Nicklaus 1974:79–80). Chris Evert rehearsed "every significant detail of an upcoming match in her mind's eye" (Lazarus 1977:68). Jean Claude Killy reported that "his only preparation for one race was to ski it mentally" (Suinn 1985:40). To be successful, a noted sports psychologist points out, such a process must not be purely imaginary but must involve a detailed kinesthetic and perceptual recreation of the performance (Suinn 1976:122). By kinesthetically refining one's concept of the desired action, the athlete is thus able to inhibit unwanted actions and facilitate the desired performance.

A number of musical performance techniques utilize a similar process of mental rehearsal, not simply to enhance performance, but as the basis for actually mastering pieces that haven't yet been learned. Bonpensierre, for instance, developed a piano technique called "ideokinesis," which avoids completely the attempt to perform a piece through physical effort, but which instead is based on waiting for the mental concept to realize itself (Bonpensiere 1953)—a process reminiscent of Zen philosophy in its focus on waiting for "It" to happen. The violinist Kreisler was said to "have memorized a concerto on the train between one big city and another, and then to have played it with the orchestra without any previous practice on the violin" (Grindea 1995:14). The importance of clear conceptualization has also been argued as the basis for vocal mastery: Kagen asserts that the key to vocal ability is not technical control of specific muscles, but a clear and accurate mental conception of the required notes (Kagen 1950:46).

Several body awareness techniques employ similar concepts for the purpose of improving bodily coordination and mobility. Dart, for instance, notes that the range of motion of the head can be affected by occluding the eye, since this facilitates the reflexes of the body that serve the need to see (Dart 1996:141). Feldenkrais employs a similar procedure by having individuals move the limb on one side and observe its range of motion. By then imagining a similar movement of the opposite limb, the subject realizes that, by simply thinking, the sensitivity and functioning of the unmoved limb has been improved (Feldenkrais 1977:136–7).

Another popular method for enhancing muscular function based on mental imagery is a technique, also called "ideokinesis," developed by Lulu Sweigard, a student of Mabel Todd. Noting that postural improvements cannot be effected through voluntary effort because they are subcortical, or involuntary, Sweigard employs mental imagery to influence reflexes. Extending Todd's technique of applying knowledge of anatomical structures to movement and coordination, Sweigard utilizes anatomical knowledge and imagery to affect muscular function at an involuntary level: "... *understanding movement,*" she wrote, "is the greatest contribution the cortex can make to effective and efficient subcortical planning of neuromuscular coordination to produce a desired movement" (Sweigard 1974:128). In various studies, Sweigard concludes that "improvement in the mechanical functions of the skeleton in weight support and movement resulted primarily from subcortical patterning of muscle function in response to the ideation involved in the process of locating and imagining movement in the body" (192). Sweigard's technique of ideokinesis is now commonly used among dancers, and graphically demonstrates the connection of mental imagery to movement.

Chiropractic and Osteopathy

Known today as a clinical and anatomically based method of spinal manipulation, chiropractic in fact has its roots in spiritualist thinking. D. D. Palmer, the founder of chiropractic, wanted to find drugless cures for disease. Influenced by the spiritualist views of the nineteenth century and dissatisfied with medical treatments, Palmer explored the ideas of Mesmer and Paracelsus, seeking to assimilate the spiritual views of harmonial thought with science while avoiding unscientific, spiritualistic vagueness. Combining the concept of laying on of hands and the manual manipulation and bone-setting techniques that dated back to Hippocrates and other ancient cultures, Palmer sought to combine "the soul cure of magnetic healing" with "the hand cure of manipulation" (Moore 1993:19).

The key to illness, according to Palmer, was subluxations, or displacements, of vertebrae, which impinge on nerves and impair conduction of nerve impulses, leading to disease. Palmer reportedly discovered the connection between spinal alignment and nerve function when, after making adjustments in a deaf patient, the patient's hearing was restored. "Nerve communications" were therefore the key to flow of life energy and good health, and the spine was central to this communication network of nerves (Moore 1993:21). By thus ensuring the proper conduction of nerve signals to various organs, the purpose of chiropractic is not to make adjustments *per se* but to restore the potential of the body to function normally.

Osteopathy, which is also a form of manipulation but which involves complete medical training, was developed by Andrew Taylor Still, an unconventional healer in the nineteenth century who, like Palmer, also sought drugless cures for disease. Similarly influenced by Mesmer and his concept of magnetic fluid and laying on of hands, Palmer stressed the centrality, not of nerve function, but of blood flow, harking back to the body humors of Greece (Waldwell 1992:30). Cranial osteopathy, a variant of osteopathy developed by William G. Sutherland, stresses the importance of adjustments to the bones of the skull.

Related to cranial osteopathy is the technique of CranioSacral Therapy developed by John Upledger. Observing that the brain and spinal cord are housed within a fluid-filled membrane which rhythmically pulses within its casing, Upledger maintains that this fluid system, which is disrupted from trauma to the skull and other causes, has a "powerful influence over a wide variety of bodily functions" (Upledger 1991:19). By restoring the ability of the bones of the skull to move and by utilizing other techniques, CranioSacral Therapy restores balance to this fluid system, resulting in a reduction of symptoms.

Bibliography

Alexander, Franz 1950. *Psychosomatic Medicine: Its Principles and Applications.* New York: W. W. Norton.

Alexander, F. Matthias 1923. *Constructive Conscious Control of the Individual.* New York: Dutton.

Alexander, F. Matthias 1910. *Man's Supreme Inheritance.* London: Methuen.

Alexander, F. Matthias 1946 (final edition, reprinted in 1996). *Man's Supreme Inheritance.* London: Mouritz.

Alexander, F. Matthias 1941. *The Universal Constant in Living.* New York: Dutton.

Alexander, F. Matthias 1932. *The Use of the Self.* New York: Dutton.

Alexander, F. Matthias 1995. *Articles and Lectures.* London: Mouritz.

Alexander, Gerda 1985. *Eutony.* New York: Felix Morrow.

Alphen, Jan Van and Anthony Aris 1996. *Oriental Medicine—An Illustrated Guide to the Asian Arts of Healing.* Boston: Shambhala.

Alster, Kristine Beyerman 1989. *The Holistic Health Movement.* Tuscaloosa: University of Alabama Press.

Aston, Judith 1991. "Your three-dimensional body—the Aston System of body usage, movement, and fitness," *Physical Therapy Today.* (Fall): 12–24.

Aston, Judith 1993. "A new approach to the dynamics of posture," *Physical Therapy Today.* 16 (3, Fall): 47–53.

Bainbridge Cohen, Bonnie 1993. *Sensing, Feeling, and Action—The Experiential Anatomy of Body-Mind Centering.* Northampton: Contact Editions.

Bartenieff, Irmgard 1980. *Body Movement—Coping with the Environment.* New York: Gordon and Breach Science Publishers.

Bartenieff, Irmgard 1995. "Functional approach to the early treatment of poliomyelitis," *Physical Therapy Review,* December, 35.

Basmajian, John V. 1967. "Control of individual motor units," *American Journal of Physical Medicine,* Vol. 46, no. 1.

Basmajian, John V. 1962. *Muscles Alive: Their Functions Revealed by Electromyography.* Baltimore: Williams and Wilkins.

Baumann, Edward, L. Piper, A. Brint, P. Wright 1978. *The Holistic Health Handbook.* Berkeley: And/Or Press.

Benson, Herbert 1975. *The Relaxation Response.* New York: William Morrow.

Bernheim, Hippolyte 1980. *Bernheim's New Studies in Hypnotism,* trans. by Richard S. Sandor. New York: International Universities Press.

Binet, Alfred 1890. *On Double Consciousness: Experimental Psychological Studies.* Chicago: Open Court.

Binet, Alfred 1890. *Alterations of Personality.* New York: D. Appleton.

Binik, Alexander 1978. "The Polarity System," from *The Holistic Health Handbook.* Berkeley: And/Or Press.

Boadella, David 1975. *Wilhelm Reich—The Evolution of His Work.* Chicago: Dell Publishing Co.

Bobath, Berta 1990. *Adult Hemiplegia: Evaluation and Treatment.* Oxford: Heinemann Medical Books.

Bobath, Berta and Karel Bobath 1975. *Motor Development in the Different Types of Cerebral Palsy.* Heinemann Medical Books.

Bonpensiere, Luigi 1953. *New Pathways to Piano Technique: A Study of the Relations Between Mind and Body with Special Reference to Piano Playing.* New York: Philosophical Library.

Braid, James 1853. "Hypnotic Therapeutics, Illustrated by Cases." Reprinted from *Monthly Journal of Medical Science,* London, 17:14–47.

Braid, James 1899. *Braid on Hypnotism.* London: George Redway.

Brett's History of Psychology 1953, ed. R. S. Peters. London: George Allen and Unwin Ltd..

Breuer, Josef and Sigmund Freud 1974. *Studies on Hysteria.* London: Penguin Books

Brown, Barbara B. 1977. *Stress and the Art of Biofeedback.* New York: Harper and Row.

Burton Goldberg Group Comp. 1993. *Alternative Medicine—The Definitive Guide.*

Cannon, Walter B. 1939. *Bodily Changes in Pain, Hunger, Fear, and Rage.* New York: D. Appleton-Century Company.

Cannon, Walter B. 1967. *The Wisdom of the Body.* New York: W. W. Norton and Company.

Carpenter, William B. 1887. *Principles of Mental Physiology, with Their Applications to the Training and Discipline of the Mind, and the Study of Its Morbid Conditions.* New York: Appleton and Co.

Caton, R. 1875. "The Electrical Currents of the Brain," *British Journal of Medicine,* 2:278.

Chopra, Deepak 1990. *Perfect Health.* New York: Harmony Books.

Chopra, Deepak 1992. *Quantum Healing.* New York: Harmony Books.

Cousins, Norman 1980. *Anatomy of an Illness.* New York: Bantam Books.

Crabtree, Adam 1993. *From Mesmer to Freud: Magnetic Sleep and the Roots of Psychological Healing.* New Haven: Yale University Press.

Dalcroze, Jacques 1921. *Rhythm, Music and Education.* New York: G. P. Putnam.

Dart, Raymond 1996. *Skill and Poise.* London: STAT Books.

Darwin, Charles 1965. *The Expression of the Emotions in Man and Animals.* Chicago: University of Chicago Press.

Das, Baba Hari and Dharma Sara Satsang 1978. "Ayurveda: The Yoga of Health," from *The Holistic Health Handbook*. Barkeley: And/Or Press.

Delacato, Carl H. 1996. *Neurological Organization and Reading.* Springfield: Charles C. Thomas.

Delacato, Carl H. 1971. *A New Start for the Child with Reading Problems.* New York: Van Rees Press.

Delacato, Carl H. 1966. *The Treatment and Prevention of Reading Problems.* Springfield: Charles C. Thomas.

Dewey, John 1957. *Human Nature and Conduct.* New York: The Modern Library.

Dimon, Theodore 1987. "Performing Arts, Pedagogy, and the Work of F. M. Alexander," Doctoral Dissertation, Harvard University.

Dimon, Theodore 1998. "The Control of Tension: A New Field for Prevention," Day Street Press.

Doman, Glenn 1974. *What to Do About Your Brain-Injured Child.* New York: private printing.

Draeger, D. and R. Smith 1980. *Comprehensive Asian Fighting Arts.* Kodansha International Ltd..

von Dürckheim, Karlfried Graf 1956. *Hara—The Vital Centre of Man.* London: George Allen & Unwin.

Eisenberg, D. 1985. *Encounters with Qi.* New York: W. W. North and Co..

Ellenberger, H. 1970. *The Discovery of the Unconscious.* New York: Basic Books.

Fay, T. 1948. "Neurophysical aspects of therapy in cerebral palsy," *Archives of Physical Medicine,* 29:327–34 (June).

Fay, T. 1955. "Origin of Human Movement," *American Journal of Psychiatry,* III:644–52 (March).

Feldenkrais, Moshe 1977. *Awareness Through Movement.* New York: Harper and Row.

Feldenkrais, Moshe 1949. *Body and Mature Behavior.* New York: International Universities Press.

Feldenkrais, Moshe 1985. *The Potent Self.* New York: Harper Collins.

Freud, Sigmund 1963. *Dora: An Analysis of a Case of Hysteria.* New York: Macmillan.

Friedman, M. and R. H. Rosenman 1971. "Type A Behavior Pattern: Its Association with Coronary Heart Disease," *Annals of Clinical Research,* 3:300–312.

Friedman, M. and R. H. Rosenman 1974. *Type A Behavior and Your Heart.* New York: Alfred A. Knopf.

Gauld, Alan 1992. *A History of Hypnotism.* Cambridge: Cambridge University Press.

Gevitz, Norman 1982. *The D.O.'s—Osteopathic Medicine in America.* Baltimore: Johns Hopkins University Press.

Gindler, E. 1986–87. "Gymnastik for Everyone," *Somatics,* vol. 6, no. I (Autumn/Winter).

Green, Elmer and Alyce Green 1977. *Beyond Biofeedback.* San Francisco: Delacorte Press.

Grindea, Carola, ed. 1995. *Tensions in the Performance of Music*. London: Kahn and Averill.

Hanna, T. 1983. *The Body of Life*. New York: Knopf.

Heller, J. and W. Henkin 1991. *Bodywise*. Berkeley: Wingbow Press.

Hengstenberg, E. 1985. *The Charlotte Selver Foundation Bulletin*. Caldwell, NJ. (Summer), 12:12.

Inglis, B. and R. West 1983. *The Alternative Health Guide*.

Jacobsen, Edmund 1938. *Progressive Relaxation*. Chicago: University of Chicago Press.

Jacobsen, Edmund 1962. *You Must Relax*. New York: McGraw-Hill.

James, William 1890a. *The Principles of Psychology*, Vol. 1. New York: Henry Holt.

James, William 1890b. *The Principles of Psychology*, Vol. 2. New York: Henry Holt.

James, William 1950. *Talks To Teachers*. New York: W. W. Norton and Co., 1958.

Janet, Pierre 1889. *L'Automatisme Psychologique: Essai de psychologie experientelle sur les formes inferieures de l'activité humaine*. Paris: Alcan.

Jones, Ernest 1953. *The Life and Work of Sigmund Freud*, Vol. 1. New York: Basic Books.

Jones, F. P. 1997. *Freedom to Change*. London: Mouritz.

Jones, F. P. 1965. "Method for changing stereotyped response patterns by the inhibition of postural sets," *Psychological Review* 72, 196–214.

Jones, W. T. 1952. *A History of Western Philosophy*. New York: Harcourt, Brace and Company.

Juhan, Deane 1984. "The Trager Approach: Psychophysical Integration and Mentastics," *The Bodywork Book*, ed. Neville Drury, Prism Alpha Press, Dorset, England.

Juhan, Deane 1987a. "The Trager Approach: A Comprehensive Introduction," *The Trager Journal*. 2 (Fall): 1–3.

Juhan, Deane 1987b. *Job's Body—A Handbook for Bodywork*. New York: Station Hill Press.

Juhan, Deane 1992. "The physiology of Hook-up: how Trager works," Keynote address, Sixth International Trager Conference, San Diego, CA. Reprint available from Trager Institute, Mill Valley, CA.

Kagen, Sergius 1950. *On Studying Singing*. New York: Dover Publications.

Kamenetz, H. L. 1980. "History of Massage," in *Manipulation, Traction, and Massage*, 2nd ed., edited by Joseph B. Rogoff, Williams and Wilkins, Baltimore.

Kamiya, J. 1968. "Conscious control of brain waves," *Psychology Today*, I: 57–60.

Kamiya, J. 1969. "Operant control of the EEG Alpha rhythm and some of its reported effects on consciousness." In C. Tart (ed.), *Altered States of Consciousness*, Julian.

Kenneson, Claude 1974. *A Cellist's Guide to the New Approach*. New York: Exposition Press.

Kraus, Hans 1974. *Backache, Stress and Tension*. New York: Pocket Book.

Laban, Rudolf 1974. *The Language of Movement: A Guidebook to Choreutics*. Annotated and edited by Lisa Ullmann. Boston: Plays.

Laban, Rudolf 1974. *Effort: Economy in Body Movement.* Boston: Plays.

Laban, Rudolf 1975. *Modern Educational Dance,* 3rd. ed., revised with additions by Lisa Ullmann. London: Macdonald and Evans.

Lazarus, A. 1977. *In the Mind's Eye.* New York: Rawson Associates.

Levine, S. 1960. "Stimulation in Infancy," *Scientific American,* May.

Levine, S. 1971. "Stress and Behavior," *Scientific American,* January.

Lindsley, D. B. 1935. "Electrical activity of human motor units during voluntary contraction," *American Journal of Physiology,* 114:90–99.

Locke, Steven 1986. *The Healer Within.* New York: Dutton.

Lowen, Alexander 1958. *The Language of the Body.* New York: Collier.

Lowen, Alexander 1976. *Bioenergetics.* New York: Penguin Books.

Luthe, W. 1962. "Method, research and application of autogenic training," *American Journal of Clinical Hypnosis,* 5, 17–23.

Magnus, R. 1925. "Animal Posture," *Proceedings of the Royal Society of London,* 98 (Ser. B), 339–53.

Magnus, R. 1924. Body Posture *(Körperstelling).* Berlin: Springer.

Magnus, R. 1926. "Physiology of Posture," *Lancet,* 211, 531–36; 585–88.

Magnus, R. 1930. "The Physiological *a priori* ," Lane lectures on experimental pharmacology and medicine: III, Stanford University Publications (Series V 2, No. 3), 331–337.

McDougall, William 1908. *Introduction to Social Psychology.* London: Methuen.

Mesmer, Franz Anton 1779. *Memoire sur la découverte du magnetisme animal.* Geneva and Paris: Didot le jeune.

Moore, J. Stuart 1993. *Chiropractic in America: The History of a Medical Alternative.* Baltimore: John Hopkins University Press.

Murphy, Gardner 1949. *Historical Introduction to Modern Psychology.* New York: Harcourt, Brace and Co.

Murphy, Michael 1993. *The Future of the Body.* Los Angeles: Jeremy Tarcher, 1993.

Nideffer, R. 1976. *The Inner Athlete.* New York: Thomas Crowell.

Nicklaus, Jack 1974. *Golf My Way.* New York: Simon and Schuster.

Pavlov, I. P. 1927. *Conditioned Reflexes: An Investigation of the Physiological Activity of the Cerebral Cortex.* London: Oxford University Press.

Pelletier, Kenneth R. 1979. *Holistic Medicine—From Stress to Optimium Health.* New York: Delacorte Press.

Pelletier, Kenneth R. 1982. *Mind as Healer, Mind as Slayer.* New York: Dell Publishing Co.

Perls, F. S. 1969. *Ego, Hunger and Aggression.* New York: Vintage Books.

Phillips, E. D. 1973. *Aspects of Greek Medicine.* New York: Thames and Hudson.

de Puységur, M. 1811. *Récherchers, experience et observations physiologiques sur l'homme dans l'état de somnambulism nature.* Paris: J. G. Dentu.

Reich, Wilhelm 1972. *Character Analysis.* New York: Farrar, Straus and Giroux.

Reich, Wilhelm 1961. *The Function of the Orgasm*. New York: Farrar, Straus and Giroux.

Reid, Daniel 1994. *The Complete Book of Chinese Health and Healing*. Boston: Shambhala.

Rolf, Ida P. 1977. *Rolfing*. New York: Harper and Row.

Rosen, M. and S. Brenner 1991. *The Rosen Method of Movement*. Berkeley: North Atlantic Books.

Rowley, David T. 1986. *Hypnosis and Hypnotherapy*. London: Croom Helm.

Rathbone, Josephine 1969. *Relaxation*. New York: Columbia University Press.

Russell, Bertrand 1945. *A History of Western Philosophy*. New York: Simon and Schuster.

Sarno, John E. 1991. *Healing Back Pain*. New York: Warner Books.

Schilder, Paul 1950. *The Image and Appearance of the Human Body*. New York: International Universities Press.

Schultz, Johannes 1960. "The clinical importance of 'inward seeing' in autogenic training," *British Journal of Medical Hypnotism*.

Schultz, J. H. and Wolfgang Luthe 1959. *Autogenic Training: A Psychophysiologic Approach in Psychotherapy*. New York: Grune and Stratton.

Selye, Hans 1956. *The Stress of Life*. New York: McGraw-Hill.

Sheldon, W. H. 1940. *The Varieties of Human Physique*. New York: Harper and Brothers.

Sheldon, W. H. 1942. *The Varieties of Temperament*. New York: Harper and Brothers.

Sherrington, C. S. 1937. *The Brain and Its Mechanism*. London: Cambridge University Press.

Sherrington, C. S. 1906. *The Endeavor of Jean Fernel*. London: Cambridge University Press.

Sherrington, C. S. 1906. *The Integrative Action of the Nervous System*. New Haven: Yale University Press.

Simonton, O. C. and S. Simonton 1975. "Belief systems and management of the emotional aspects of malignancy," *Journal of Transpersonal Psychology,* 7, No. 1: 29–47.

Simonton, O. C. and S. Simonton 1978. *Getting Well Again*. Los Angeles: Jeremy Tarcher.

Smith, Frederick 1986. *Inner Bridges—A Guide to Energy Movement and Body Structure*. Atlanta: Humanics, New Age.

Smith, Olive 1934. "Action Potentials from Single Motor Units in Voluntary Contraction," *American Journal of Physiology,* 108:629–38.

Spencer, Herbert 1899. *Principles of Psychology*. New York: D. Appleton and Co.

Stone, R. 1948. *The Vital Principle in the Healing Art*. Chicago: private printing.

Suinn, R. 1976. "Body thinking: psychology for olympic athletes," *Psychology Today* (July), 10:38–43.

Suinn, R. 1985. "Imagery rehearsal: application to performance enhancement," *Behavior Therapist,* 8: 155–59.

Suzuki, D. T. 1959. *Zen and Japanese Culture.* Princeton: Princeton University Press, Bollingen Series.

Sweigard, Lulu E. 1974. *Human Movement Potential.* New York: Harper and Row.

Thorndike, E. 1905. *The Elements of Psychology.* New York: A. G. Seiler.

Tinbergen, Niko 1972. "The Croonian Lecture," *Proc. R. Soc. Lond. B.* 182, 385–410.

Tinbergen, Niko 1974. "Ethology and Stress Disease," *Science,* July, Vol. 185, 20–27.

Todd, Mabel E. 1953. *The Hidden You.* New York: Dance Horizons.

Todd, Mabel E. 1937. *The Thinking Body.* New York: Dance Horizons.

Trager, Milton and C. Guadagno 1987. *Trager Mentastics: Movement as a Way to Agelessness.* Barrytown, New York: Station Hill Press.

Upledger, John E. 1991. *Your Inner Physician and You.* Berkeley: North Atlantic Books.

Waldwell, W. 1992. *Chiropractors: History and Evolution of a New Profession.* St. Louis: Mosby-Year Book.

Wallace, R. K. 1970. "Physiological effects of Transcendental Meditation," *Science,* 167:1751–54.

Wallace, R. K. and H. Benson 1972. "The physiology of meditation," *Scientific American,* 226:84–90.

Watson, J. B. 1925. *Behaviorism.* New York: W. W. Norton.

White, John and James Fadiman, eds. 1976. *Relax.* New York: Dell Books.

Wolpe, J. 1974. *The Practice of Behavior Therapy.* New York: Pergamon.

Wolpe, J. 1958. *Psychotherapy by Reciprocal Inhibition.* Stanford: Stanford University Press.

Woodall, Percy H. 1920. *Osteopathy—The Science of Healing by Adjustment.* Orange, New Jersey: American Osteopathic Association.

Worthington, Vivian 1982. *A History of Yoga.* London: Routledge and Kegan Paul.

Index